Study Guide to ~

Kemp, Pillitteri, and Brown's

FUNDAMENTALS OF NURSING

Study Guide to Accompany

Kemp, Pillitteri, and Brown's

FUNDAMENTALS OF NURSING: A FRAMEWORK FOR PRACTICE

Second Edition

Patricia Brown, Ph.D., R.N.C.
Associate Professor, Marion A. Buckley School of Nursing
Adelphi University, Garden City, New York

Sheila Gettelson, Ed.D., R.N.
Assistant Professor, Marion A. Buckley School of Nursing
Adelphi University, Garden City, New York

Jean Winter, Ed.D., R.N.
Assistant Professor, Marion A. Buckley School of Nursing
Adelphi University, Garden City, New York

Scott, Foresman/Little, Brown College Division

SCOTT, FORESMAN AND COMPANY

Glenview, Illinois   Boston   London

ISBN 0-673-39794-7

1 2 3 4 5 6 7 8 9 10—VIK—94 93 92 91 90 89 88

Printed in the United States of America

TO THE STUDENT

This Study Guide is designed to help you assimilate and master the basic nursing concepts and techniques presented in the text *Fundamentals of Nursing: A Framework for Practice,* Second Edition, by Kemp, Pillitteri, and Brown. Used as a supplement, this guide emphasizes the most important aspects of each chapter and provides an avenue for self-assessment, reinforcement of learning, and application of knowledge.

The chapters in this Study Guide correspond to the text chapters. Each chapter includes the following sections:

- *Major Nursing Concepts.* This section summarizes and highlights the major concepts presented in each text.

- *Drill and Practice Questions for Review.* A variety of drill and practice questions are presented to help you identify topics that you may need to study further. Question format is varied to make this process more interesting. Short-answer questions include completion and true/false items and matching columns as well as case situations with related questions. These will challenge you to apply your new knowledge in real-life scenarios relevant to the content area of particular chapters. Many situations require you to demonstrate professional judgment in implementation of the nursing process.

- *Answers to Drill and Practice Questions.* Answers are provided for **all** Drill and Practice questions, including the situations, for each chapter.

Here's to your success in mastering the *Fundamentals of Nursing!*

P.B.
S.G.
J.W.

CONTENTS

Study Guide to Accompany

Kemp, Pillitteri, and Brown's

FUNDAMENTALS OF NURSING

PART I

INTRODUCTION TO NURSING PRACTICE

Chapter 1

THE PROFESSION OF NURSING

MAJOR NURSING CONCEPTS

Nursing care of people is a practice that is as old as humankind. In early times, nursing care was usually performed by close relatives.

Hippocrates who is referred to as the "Father of Medicine," emphasized the need for accurate observations and recording. Those who assisted him, such as priests and male nurses, were better educated and better informed than was the average citizen.

During the Middle Ages, nursing care was performed by both men and women in hospitals affiliated with convents and monasteries. Nursing education consisted of a one-year apprenticeship with practicing nurses.

During the Reformation, convent and monastery hospitals were closed. Because these orders were involved in health care, nursing and hospital care suffered. When nursing orders were restored, they were located in government-sponsored hospitals and primarily hired women. As more and more women entered nursing, it became a profession synonymous with women.

The English nurse **Florence Nightingale** is notable for having moved nurses and the profession of nursing into an era of respectability by organizing and upgrading nursing education and nursing practice. Nursing care at that time was performed by **caring, knowledgeable,** and **loyal women** who were learning to base their nursing activities on scientific reasoning.

At the time of World War II, nurses were beginning to make **independent judgments** and to assume more responsibility, resulting in a public recognition of them as individuals capable of delivering safe and effective nursing care.

Nurse practice acts are established by legislative bodies in each state in order to define nursing and the boundaries of nursing practice.

Modern nursing care is built upon a **unique body of knowledge** that has steered nursing practice away from not only the medical model but also the image of physician's assistant and handmaiden. Nursing practice today focuses on **health promotion, prevention, and maintenance and restoration of health.** Nurses are teachers, nurturers, comforters, planners, coordinators, and advocates. They are involved in total client care.

Nursing theory is knowledge that is specific to nursing. Nurse theorists try to explain systematically the general principles which underlie and guide nursing practice. According to Nightingale, actions should be directed toward changing an individual's environment. **Henderson** believes that there are fourteen basic needs with which nurses can assist clients in order to help the clients toward greater independence. **Orem** states that nursing is guided by the individual's ability for self-care.

The International Council of Nurses (ICN) is a worldwide organization that serves as a resource center for nursing knowledge in order to strengthen and improve nursing care.

The American Nurses Association (ANA) is one of many professional nursing organizations in the United States. Its activities include the promotion and improvement of health care; the maintenance of high standards for professional education; and the professional development of nurses throughout the country.

Both the ICN and the ANA have published a Code of Ethics for nursing practice, which is discussed fully in Chapter 5.

The question of whether nursing is a true profession is frequently debated. **A true profession has the following characteristics:** it is practice based on a well-defined body of theoretical knowledge; it provides a necessary human service; and it has autonomy (self-regulation) in practice, with members practicing under a specific code of ethics.

Standards of Nursing Practice have been developed by the ANA to help maintain a high level of nursing practice. They are organized according to the five steps of the nursing process; assessment, analysis, planning of care, implementation, and evaluation of care.

The ANA's position paper on nursing education (1965) states that nursing education should take place in schools of higher learning (colleges and universities). Basic education for individuals seeking to be registered nurses presently occurs in three kinds of programs: baccalaureate, associate degree, and diploma programs. Programs differ in philosophy as well as in the skills and knowledge base of the graduates. Nontraditional nursing education programs, which exist for mature, independent learners, are geared to content areas rather than classroom attendance. Continuing education programs, such as those leading to master's and doctorate degrees, are available to people interested in specializing in the areas of education, administration, and research.

The **1985 New York State Nurses Association Resolution** proposes that the entry level for beginning professional nursing practice be at the baccalaureate level. The associate nurse would be educated in a diploma program or in a college granting an associate degree. Previously licensed graduates would be "grandfathered" in and would retain the title of professional nurse.

Certification is granted by professional nursing organizations to nurses who demonstrate a high level of nursing knowledge. Certification in a specialty area can lead to promotion and salary increase.

The **National Student Nurses Association (NSNA)** is an organization open to all undergraduate nursing students. NSNA activities include programs that assist students in the development of a professional role.

Nurses today can practice in a variety of roles (clinical nurse specialist, consultant, researcher, author) and in a variety of settings (industry, clinics, schools, homes, hospitals). Hospitals are acute care facilities which employ the largest number of nurses. A patient's length of stay in a hospital is usually short. Clients in need of extended health-care services can be transferred to convalescent, chronic care facilities. Nurses working in community settings are usually

Public Health nurses employed by the state, county, or local health department. Total health care in the community may involve teaching people how to care for themselves or for family members recently discharged from a hospital.

Nurses with advanced education and/or experience can practice in expanded roles (nurse practitioner, clinical nurse specialist, consultant, researcher).

DRILL AND PRACTICE QUESTIONS FOR REVIEW

Complete the statements below.

1. _____ is frequently referred to as the Father of Medicine.

2. Florence Nightingale moved the nursing profession into an era of respectability by _____.

3. _____ legally define nursing with regulations guiding practice.

4. The person who tries to explain systematically the principles that guide nursing practice is referred to as a _____.

5. Changing the patient's environment in order to assist him or her in the recovery process is a theory by _____.

6. Assisting people with their fourteen basic needs when they cannot provide them for themselves is a concept developed by _____.

7. Orem's theory of nursing is called _____.

8. Three functions of the American Nurses Association are _____, _____, and _____.

9. Three characteristics of a profession are _____, _____, and _____.

10. The organization that speaks for nurses worldwide is the _____.

Determine whether the following statements are TRUE or FALSE.

1. Members of a profession have control over issues of practice.

2. Today's nurse practices from a nursing model that focuses on disease.

3. Nursing practice is guided by the American Medical Association and the Hospital Association.

4. Ethical standards of practice developed by the American Nurses Association and the International Council of Nurses set standards for nursing practice.

5. The nursing process consists of these five steps: assessment, analysis, planning, implementation, and evaluation.

6. Information gained by assessment should not be communicated to the entire health care team.

7. Nursing diagnoses are based on nursing problems.

8. In the planning of patient care, goals should be determined with the client and stated in realistic, measurable terms.

9. Setting priorities for care enables the nurse to meet the patient's most serious needs first.

10. Nursing actions should be based on traditional practices.

11. The entry level for professional nursing practice should be at the associate degree level.

12. There are differences in state licensure between diploma, associate degree, and baccalaureate graduates.

13. Continuing education requirements for license renewal is standard throughout the country.

14. Membership in professional nursing organizations is mandatory upon graduation from nursing school.

ANSWERS TO DRILL AND PRACTICE QUESTIONS

Complete the statements below.

1. Hippocrates

2. improving the training of nurses

3. nurse practice acts

4. nurse theorist

5. Nightingale

6. Henderson

7. universal self-care

8. The promotion and improvement of health standards; access to health care services for all and the maintenance of high standards for professional education.

9. that it is a practice based on a well-defined body of theoretical knowledge; that it provides a needed human service; and that it has autonomy guided by a code of ethics.

10. International Council of Nurses

True/False Exercises

1.	T	8.	T
2.	F	9.	T
3.	F	10.	F
4.	T	11.	F
5.	T	12.	F
6.	F	13.	F
7.	F	14.	F

Chapter 2

THE NURSING ROLE IN THE HEALTH CARE DELIVERY SYSTEM

MAJOR NURSING CONCEPTS

Health care is considered a **basic, universal health right.**

The **health care delivery system** can be defined as the manner in which health care is provided to people. In the United States, health care is the second largest business. Its goals include health maintenance (promotion of health and the prevention of illness); health restoration (acute and long term care); and assistance toward accepted death with dignity. The kinds of health care offered and access to the health care delivery system are influenced by government commitment and spending as well as the age; knowledge level, life style, culture, attitudes, and values of the population.

Comprehensive health care provides the patient with total, individualized, patient-centered care. All individuals, including nurses and doctors, are potential consumers of health care.

Morbidity refers to the yearly incidence of disease or illness. **Mortality** refers to the number of deaths per year, per one thousand people. The infant mortality rate is the criterion for determining the effectiveness of health care throughout the world.

Providers of health care include **official agencies** supported by tax dollars (World Health Organization, Health and Human Services, Food and Drug Administration, Centers for Disease Control, National Institute for Health, and the Health Services Agency) and **voluntary agencies** supported by private funds (private nonprofit hospitals, private profit-making hospitals, and private organizations like the American Heart Association). The purposes of the federal Health Services Agency (HSA) are to restrain rising health costs, prevent unnecessary repetition of health services, and improve existing health care services.

Health care services are differentiated according to the levels of preventive activities used. **Primary prevention and care,** which centers on health promotion, is geared to keeping people well. Educational material from a local heart association on reducing the risks of heart attack with exercise and good nutrition are examples of primary prevention strategies. The American Heart Association is an example of a primary prevention agency. **Secondary prevention and care** includes early diagnosis and treatment of illness. This level may also refer to caring for a patient after surgery. Hospitals and ambulatory care facilities are examples of secondary prevention care facilities. **Tertiary prevention and care** focuses on rehabilitation. This level of care may involve a nurse teaching a stroke victim how to walk and talk. Nursing homes and agencies that focus on helping the handicapped are examples of tertiary prevention care agencies.

Diagnostic Related Groups (DRGs) comprise a patient classification system set up by the federal Medicare system to curb the high cost of health care. As a result, hospitalized patients are being discharged earlier than ever before, many of whom have unresolved health care problems. In effect only a few years, this system has dramatically changed nursing priorities for care in secondary and tertiary agencies.

5

Health Maintenance Organizations (HMOs) are systems that offer unlimited comprehensive health care. For a fee, members can avail themselves of unlimited health care services. The focus of this plan is primary prevention or maintenance of wellness. Nurses play an active role in the delivery of this type of health care. **Preferred Provider Organizations** contract with employers to provide health care to employees. This type of health care plan is similar to the HMO except that it terminates at the end of employment.

Hospice care involves supportive physical and emotional care to those who are prepared for and have accepted impending death. The physiological, psychological, and emotional care provided is comprehensive, and it involves not only the patient but also the patient's family and/or significant other.

Consumers of health care can pay for health services by personal payment (cash or check); voluntary insurance (Blue Cross, Blue Shield), or social insurance (Medicare, Medicaid, or Workmen's Compensation).

Problems with the health-care delivery system are likely to arise from its size, lack of planning, emphasis on illness care, poor allocation of services, or lack of consumer interest or input into decision making.

Quality Assurance Programs and Professional Standard Review Organization were both established to set standards of health care and to monitor the health care delivery system against specific standards. The Joint Commission on Accreditation of Hospitals (JCAH) is a voluntary, nonprofit organization that monitors health care agencies for quality of care. Health care agencies receive reimbursement (Medicare or Medicaid) for services only if they are accredited by the JCAH.

The nurse's role in the health care delivery system is diversified. The nurse of today is educated to function in various settings and in cooperation with other health care personnel.

DRILL AND PRACTICE QUESTIONS FOR REVIEW

Complete the statements below.

1. The second largest industry in the United States is _____.
2. Comprehensive health care provides the patient with _____.
3. Morbidity may be defined as _____.
4. Activities of the Health Services Agency include _____, _____, and _____.
5. The Food and Drug Administration is responsible for _____.
6. The World Health Organization is responsible for _____ and _____.
7. The federal agency concerned with the incidence of health problems and ways to protect people against outbreaks of illnesses is the _____.
8. Primary prevention is aimed at _____.
9. Children born with a birth defect are placed into a _____ prevention level of care.
10. Medicare provides for health services for people over the age of _____.
11. The purpose of Diagnostic Related Groups is to _____.

6

12. The major purpose of quality assurance programs in institutions is to _____.

13. A community hospital is an example of a _____ agency.

14. A young child being immunized against diphtheria is receiving care at the _____ prevention level.

15. The purpose of the Professional Standard Review organization is to _____.

16. The ultimate focus of hospice care is to _____.

17. Four ways nurses can promote better health care are _____, _____, _____, and _____.

Determine whether the following statements are TRUE or FALSE.

1. The goals of a modern health care delivery system include health maintenance and health restoration.

2. Health restoration includes acute care and long term care.

3. Health care throughout the world is standardized.

4. Nurses should be aware of health related issues and actively support legislators sympathetic to health related issues.

5. Community health care programs are usually successful if a community assessment is done.

6. The United States has a very low infant mortality rate.

7. The National Institute for Health includes a new center for nursing research.

8. Secondary prevention and care includes early diagnosis of acute conditions.

9. Tertiary prevention and care includes rehabilitation and assisting the patient toward maximum potential.

10. Educating the public about risks of heart disease is an example of primary prevention.

11. Patients who are discharged early because of diagnostic related groups (DRGs) do not need health instruction.

12. Health Maintenance Organizations (HMOs) are examples of Episodic Care Centers.

13. The system by which hospitals are reimbursed a predetermined amount of money for categories of health care is called Medicaid.

14. Because of diagnostic related groups, patients in the home tend to be sicker and require skilled nursing care.

ANSWERS TO DRILL AND PRACTICE QUESTIONS

Completion Exercises

1. health care

2. total, individualized, patient-centered care

3. yearly incidence of illness or disease

4. preventing repetition of health services and restraining rising health care cost, and improving existing health care services

5. enforcing laws related to drugs, food, and cosmetics

6. promoting better care in health and related professions; providing information, counseling, and help in the area of health care; and promoting and conducting health research

7. Centers for Disease Control

8. health promotion, or keeping people well

9. secondary

10. 65

11. curb the increasing cost of health care

12. provide the public with a high standard of care

13. local level, nonprofit

14. primary prevention

15. decide whether health care agencies supported by Medicare and Medicaid are safe and economical, and meet professional standards

16. assist individuals toward a painless death with dignity

17. initiate new ideas based on research; take active role in health planning; support legislators active in promoting health; be aware of consumer needs; encourage clients to take an active role in their health care; consider cost effective procedures; individualize and coordinate care

True/False Exercises

1.	T	8.	T
2.	T	9.	T
3.	F	10.	T
4.	T	11.	F
5.	T	12.	F
6.	F	13.	F
7.	T	14.	T

PART II

CONCEPTUAL FOUNDATIONS OF NURSING PRACTICE

Chapter 3

CONSUMER RIGHTS AND HEALTH CARE

NOTE TO STUDENT

The Patient's Bill of Rights, along with the nursing implications, are discussed in detail throughout this chapter.

Nurses' Rights are highlighted in box fashion in this chapter.

MAJOR NURSING CONCEPTS

The main purpose of the American Hospital Association's **Bill of Rights** is to inform patients about what they should expect from their physicians and hospitals during hospitalization. This Bill of Rights also applies to individuals receiving home health care. A separate Bill of Rights protects clients who are elderly, dying, handicapped, mentally retarded, mentally ill, or pregnant. This information is usually given to the patient or a family member at the time of hospital admission. Although the document is not legally binding in most states, following the guidelines is required of all hospitals seeking accreditation by the Joint Commission on Accreditation of Hospitals (JCAH). These guidelines have strong implications for nursing, since nurses are the prime caregivers. In order to provide quality health care, nurses should follow the standards listed in the patient's Bill of Rights as well as those in the American Nurses Association's Code of Ethics (discussed in Chapter 3).

A **client advocate** is employed by the health care agency and tries to ensure patient rights. The advocate may also represent a client whose rights have been violated (a client has the right to know about and should be informed about his or her illness, procedures, and medications). The client advocate, who may be a nurse, supports the individual in making the best possible decision concerning his or her health care. When nurses are advocates (attempting to assist clients with problems), they must observe the lines of authority in the health care agency.

Nurses have rights. These rights can be safeguarded if nurses join their professional associations, especially the American Nurses Association—Nurses Coalition for Action in Politics (N—CAP). In addition, by keeping informed about legislation directly affecting their profession and about legislators who are sympathetic to their problems as nurses, nurses can keep their rights secure. It is also important for nurses to know whether their employers recognize, accept, and support the Nurses' Bill of Rights.

9

DRILL AND PRACTICE QUESTIONS FOR REVIEW

Complete the statements below.

1. The American Hospital Association's Bill of Rights asserts the rights of _____.

2. Before any procedure can be performed on a patient, _____ must be obtained.

3. The statement, "the right to refuse treatment to the extent permitted by law," is from the _____.

4. Standards of Care are achievable levels of _____.

5. Jehovah's Witnesses may refuse _____.

6. International safeguards for children are stated in the United Nations _____.

7. The Rights of Handicapped Persons state that they _____ and _____.

8. Health care to the mentally retarded must protect their rights in the area of _____.

Determine whether the following statements are TRUE or FALSE.

1. Hospitalized patients should expect up-to-date information related to their illness and treatment.

2. A Spanish-speaking client should not expect information concerning his illness to be given to him in Spanish.

3. Respectful care includes consideration of developmental needs and age differences.

4. Prognosis refers to the prospect of recovery from an illness.

5. Informed consent is not a legal requirement before a special procedure is done to a hospitalized patient.

6. Discussing a patient's condition in a public elevator violates the patient's right to privacy.

7. Hospitalized clients do not have the right to see an itemized bill of health care services performed.

8. Hospitalized clients do not have to be asked if they want to participate in a research study.

9. Nurse's aides, hospital attendants, and volunteers have their own code of professional ethics.

10. When acting as a client advocate, the nurse goes directly to the Director of Nursing with the problem.

11. The Code of Ethics and the Patient's Bill of Rights are legally enforceable documents.

Situations

Situation 1

As a nursing student caring for Mrs. Green, you learn that she is going to have surgery this morning. Mrs. Green tells you that she does not understand why she needs the operation nor what risks are involved. What would be an appropriate nursing action at this time?

10

Situation 2

When you are in the local supermarket, you hear hospital volunteers discussing one of your patients. They are talking loudly about his diagnosis, prognosis, and test results. What would be appropriate for you to do at this time?

ANSWERS TO DRILL AND PRACTICE QUESTIONS

Completion Exercises

1. patients concerning their health care

2. informed consent

3. Patient's Bill of Rights

4. behavior/performance

5. blood transfusions

6. Declaration of the Rights of the Child

7. must not be discriminated against trying to enter schools, public buildings; health care institutions and interpreters must be available if communication problems affect safe health care practices

8. informed consent

True/False Exercises

1. T		6.	T
2. F		7.	F
3. T		8.	F
4. T		9.	F
5. F		10.	F
		11.	F

Situations

Situation 1

The nurse should notify the physician scheduled to do the surgery of the patient's lack of understanding of the impending procedure. It is the physician's responsibility to inform the patient about the procedure, including the risks involved and available alternatives. When the patient communicates understanding of the proposed surgery (its risks and alternatives), the elements of Informed Consent have been achieved.

Situation 2

The volunteers must be reminded that any discussion of patients is inappropriate and violates the Patient's Bill of Rights.

Chapter 4

LEGAL ASPECTS OF NURSING PRACTICE

MAJOR NURSING CONCEPTS

Laws are rules made by society in order to control conduct.

Legislative laws (**nurse practice acts**) originate with a government body. The nursing profession is governed by the legislative body of each state.

Common law, which developed from English tradition, is referred to as precedent or judicial law. Common-law decisions have implications for nursing as new procedures and different nursing roles emerge.

Criminal laws, which protect the safety and property of citizens, include crimes such as felonies (murders, robberies) and misdemeanors (assaults, motor vehicle violations).

Civil laws focus on private rights. **Torts** are violations of civil law which result in serious inconvenience or harm to the individual. Nurses are most often involved in civil actions, such as offenses against individuals (patients).

Professional misconduct (violations of practice) is defined and determined by individual State Boards of Nursing. Nurses found guilty of major professional misconduct (practicing beyond the scope of their nurse practice act, theft of drugs, mental incompetence) are subject to license suspension or revocation by the individual State Boards of Nursing. Alcohol and drug abuse are the most frequent problems facing nurses, nursing, and State Boards of Nursing today.

The **nurse-patient relationship** is a special, binding relationship that nurses must seriously and conscientiously honor. Once this relationship begins (verbally or nonverbally), it is the nurse's legal responsibility to continue or supervise quality care until properly replaced by another health care provider. **Abandonment** is the act of terminating patient care after the nurse-patient relationship had been established. Should harm occur to the patient during the nurse's absence, legal action (civil action, criminal lawsuit, suspension or loss of nursing license) could follow. At the time of their employment, nurses should notify employers if they have religious or ethical beliefs that prevent them from caring for patients with certain types of problems.

Respondent Superior is a Latin term meaning "let the master answer." It has implications for nursing because it implies that the employer (hospital) is responsible for the health care delivered by its employees (nurses). However, nurses can be held liable if they do not practice within the scope of their nurse practice act or do not follow hospital procedure and policy. Even with the doctrine of Respondent Superior, nursing students, practicing nurses, and nursing instructors are still legally responsible for their own actions. The doctrine of Respondent Superior also implies that nurses are responsible for appropriately delegating patient care to personnel assigned to them.

Negligence is the omission (leaving ice on a private walkway) or commission (keeping fire exits locked) of an act that a reasonable person would or would not do. It applies to all people. **Contributory negligence** occurs when a patient participates in her own injury (if after receiving a sedative and instructions to remain in bed, the patient gets out of the bed, falls, and injures herself).

Malpractice is the negligent act of a professional person (nurse, lawyer, physician). Three criteria are necessary for a malpractice suit: nursing error, patient injury, and a direct relationship between the two (proximate cause). It is the patient's responsibility to prove that malpractice has occurred. Specific guidelines that may be used to determine whether a nurse practiced in the way that another reasonable and prudent nurse would act in the same situation include the following: Standards of Practice, Nurse Practice Acts, the nurse's level of education and knowledge, the health care agency's policy and procedure book, job descriptions, patient's Bill of Rights, expert witnesses, current texts, and current periodicals.

Nurse practice Acts, which vary from state to state, identify the full legal scope of nursing practice. In addition, Standards of Care established by the American Nurses' Association are accepted guidelines for nursing practice. Nurses are at risk for legal action if they practice outside either one of these guidelines. High-risk nursing practice activities that can adversely affect patient safety and possibly incur a malpractice suit include medication administration; application of heat and cold; use of new, unfamiliar equipment; moving and ambulating clients; inadequate health teaching; and poor verbal and written communication skills.

Nurses are responsible for the psychological and physiological safety of patients entrusted to their care. Administration of an injection without consent (assault); holding a patient for nonpayment of a hospital bill (false imprisonment); securing a patient indefinitely to the bed with restraints without a physician's order; disregarding a patient's right to refuse care; violation of confidentiality and privacy; and defamation of character (a written derogatory statement is libel; a verbal derogatory statement is slander) are problem areas directly related to patient safety and can constitute a cause for legal action against the nurse. In general, malpractice suits against nurses have been instituted when patients are unhappy with their care and when nurses are impersonal, discourteous, not knowledgeable, and unsafe, and when nurses demonstrate a level of practice lacking care and concern for the patient. Patients also institute lawsuits when they are stressed, have poor prognosis, and have not received adequate, accurate health teaching upon discharge from the institution.

Good Samaritan Laws protect health care providers from legal action when giving emergency care outside the health care delivery system. As long as health care personnel provide reasonable care under the circumstances, they should not be held responsible for poor outcomes.

People have the right to refuse health care. People have the right to make a decision about their health care based on accurate, up-to-date information. People have the right to sign a consent specifying the care they choose to receive. This consent, in order to be legal, must be informed. Informed consent consists of an explanation of the proposed procedure, related risks, and alternatives to the proposed procedure. This document provides the patient with information on which to make a knowledgeable decision about health care. A consent is not considered informed if the patient was sedated or if the information was so technical that the patient could not understand the language. Informed consent is not necessary for life-saving procedures such as cardiopulmonary resuscitation.

Incident reports are documents describing potential or actual injury to patient, staff, or visitors. Incident reports are not part of the patient's medical record and should not be mentioned when writing about the incident or injury in the patient's record. The information contained in the incident report should describe the error, whether an injury occurred to the patient, and what the relationship was between the two (proximal cause). This form also serves to prevent future injury by recognizing the cause of the incident and instituting corrective measures.

DRILL AND PRACTICE QUESTIONS FOR REVIEW

Complete the statements below.

1. Three acts that may cause a nurse to have her or his license suspended are _____, _____, and _____.

2. _____ is the act of leaving a patient without continuing health care.

3. The phrase _____ _____ implies that an employer is responsible for the actions of employees.

4. The term _____ can be applied when a nurse does not act in accordance with professional standards of care.

5. Three criteria of informed consent are _____, _____, and _____.

6. High-risk areas of nursing practice include _____, _____, and _____.

7. The suit-prone nurse is usually one who is _____ and _____.

8. Failure to use restraints properly on a hospitalized patient is an example of a _____.

Match the definitions with the terms:

1. _____ assault
2. _____ battery
3. _____ civil law

4. _____ Good Samaritan Laws
5. _____ libel
6. _____ malpractice
7. _____ negligence

8. _____ slander

a. written defamatory statements

b. includes felonies

c. omission/commission of an act that a reasonable person would/ would not do

d. negligence at a professional level

e. spoken derogatory statement

f. threat of harm

g. concerned with offenses against individuals

h. touching of another without consent

i. protects health care personnel from legal action when giving emergency care

True/False Exercises

1. Licensing of nurses takes place at a national level.

2. Torts are violations of civil law resulting in injury.

3. Drug and alcohol abuse are the most common offenses associated with professional misconduct.

4. Student nurses are not liable for their actions in the clinical setting.

5. Private duty nurses are regarded as independent contractors and should carry their own malpractice insurance.

6. It is not necessary for nurses to be familiar with policies and procedures of health care agencies in which they practice.

7. All nurses are expected to perform at the same level of practice regardless of different levels of educational preparation.

8. Hospital administration may choose not to defend a nurse whose actions were outside her job description.

9. Clients should expect that health care personnel should be knowledgeable, caring, and kind.

Situation

As the nurse in charge of many patients on a unit, you assigned a new, inexperienced nursing assistant to care for a very sick woman who was having a blood transfusion. The aide had no previous experience caring for either a very sick patient or a patient receiving a blood transfusion. During this nurse's aides care, the patient fell out of bed, resulting in the blood transfusion becoming dislodged. Discuss the legal issues involved in this situation.

ANSWERS TO DRILL AND PRACTICE QUESTIONS

Completion Exercises

1. alcohol/drug abuse; working without a renewed license; prescribing medications

2. abandonment

3. respondent superior

4. malpractice

5. explanation of procedure, risks, and alternatives

6. medication administration, application of heat and cold, transfer, and ambulation

7. discourteous, unsafe, not knowledgeable

8. negligent nursing action

Matching

1. f
2. h
3. g
4. i

5. a
6. d
7. c
8. e

True/False Exercises

1.	F	6.	F
2.	T	7.	F
3.	T	8.	F
4.	F	9.	T
5.	T	10.	F

Situation

The doctrine of Respondent Superior implies that the nurse, as a representative of the hospital, is legally responsible for the actions of the aide. It is as if she herself had provided the care, and thus she can be sued for malpractice. The nurse should have been aware of the job description, knowledge, and experience level of the aide before assigning her a patient requiring care beyond the aide's capabilities.

Chapter 5

ETHICAL ASPECTS OF NURSING PRACTICE

NOTE TO STUDENT

The American Nurses' Association Code of Ethics is discussed fully in this chapter.

Guidelines for Ethical Decision Making are listed and discussed in the Focus on Nursing 2-1 of this chapter.

MAJOR NURSING CONCEPTS

Laws are enforceable rules made by society in order to control conduct. They are designed to protect the safety and rights of individuals.

Ethics are moral principles or values that people should follow so that their behavior is considered morally proper. Ethical rules incorporate a caring attitude towards others. The nursing profession has established its own Code of Ethics for nursing practice.

Ethical Development takes place across the life span and differs greatly because of religious, cultural, social, and family influences. Nurses need to be very aware of the natural differences that exist in the beliefs and value systems of the patients whom they care for. Understanding the values and beliefs of other people enables the nurse to care for clients without expecting them to alter or change their beliefs to fit the standards of the caregiver.

Ethical Behavior is learned in early childhood. It reflects the actions of parents based on the value system stressed in the home.

Infant. Children under three years of age have little understanding of right or wrong. Their behavior is geared to pleasing the caregiver.

Toddler and Preschooler. The child learns mostly by touching and feeling. The behavior of the child reflects the yes or no response of the caregiver. The child begins to develop a conscience at preschool level. It is at this time that the child begins to learn that he or she may not perform certain actions, not because the actions are right or wrong but because of the punishment that may result

School-ager and Adolescent. The school-ager begins to form his or her own personal values and standards. It is also at this time that the child begins to do unkind things to other children. The adolescent begins to form a personal identity, in terms of which ethical standards will guide his or her behavior. As the adolescent strives for independence, he or she tends to view values and beliefs quite differently from the parents. The adolescent is also learning how to use adult reasoning in ethical decision making. He or she is learning that it is wrong to perform a certain act not because of the punishment that may result but because it may cause harm to another person. This represents beginning decision making capabilities with internal control.

17

Adulthood. Young adulthood is a time of image and identity building. Although the values, attitudes, or beliefs of the young adult do not change dramatically over time, they can be modified. As young adults move into middle and older age, however, values and ethical standards tend to become more fixed. As discussed before, many professions, like nursing, have a code of ethics. Young adults working in health care agencies may find that their personal codes of ethics conflict with those of the professional organization. Working in a health care agency, the young adult may find that it is very difficult to care for a patient who has had an abortion or to care for a patient who has received an organ transplant.

Values are in depth, deeply rooted, freely chosen qualities or convictions that reflect life experiences and that relate strongly to one's personal identity. A value system can be so strong that the individual will do anything to defend it. Values differ from needs, beliefs, or interests.

According to **Abraham Maslow,** there is a **hierarchy of needs** that determines and influences the actions of individuals. They do not usually reflect values because independent decision making or free choice is not involved. Needs are strong, internal feelings (tensions) generated by some change in the individual or the individual's environment. The uneasiness or tension results in specific behaviors (goal-directed) which are focused on reducing that intense feeling or tension and on meeting that need.

> *First-level.* Air, food, water, sleep, and activity are basic physiological needs that people want to have met first.
>
> *School-level.* Protection, safety, security, and freedom from fear, anxiety, and harm are needs that emerge after first-level needs have been met.
>
> *Third-level.* Love, sense of belonging, friends, and a sense that one is loved are needs that emerge after the second-level needs have been met.
>
> *Fourth-level.* Self esteem, liking and respecting oneself are needs that center around the person's self-identity and a feeling of self-worth.
>
> *Fifth-level.* Feeling truly fulfilled as an individual and reaching the point of knowing that personal goals have been reached is the highest achievement.

Interests and feelings guide behavior; however, they are usually at a more superficial level than are values. This placement occurs because they frequently reflect current, temporary situations rather than in depth, deeply rooted persuasions based on life experiences.

Beliefs are attitudes or patterns of thought that an individual has gained throughout a lifetime. Because beliefs do not reflect the concept of free choice and because they have been with the individual for a very long time. The term *beliefs* should not be used interchangeably with *values*.

Personal values develop from life experiences and from interactions and interplay of family, friends, sex, religion, community, country, and culture. Personal values may include items such as paintings, but may also include an idea of worth such as honesty. Values are important to people because they are prized, and their loss may cause sorrow. Values are influenced by age, life experiences, and environmental influences. They are not constant in nature but are modified or changed during one's life.

Environment influences affect personal values in very special ways. For example, the depression of the 1930s made people realize that financial security should be a high priority. Another example is the trend toward married couples' delaying having children. Financial security and personal career goals have supplanted traditional desires for having children early in a marriage.

Situational influences along with environmental influences affect changing value systems. Situational influences may include changing life styles, the need for permanent rather than temporary housing, and personal health status.

A professional code of ethics is found in most professions. The nursing profession has established its specific guidelines for ethical behavior in nursing practice via the American Nurses' Association and the International Council of Nurses. Although these guidelines are neither established by law nor legally binding, failing to follow them may be cause for a state board of nursing to suspend a license or for an employer to terminate employment.

Ethical problems in nursing practice usually develop when there is a conflict between what the nurse believes ought to be done, what the Nursing Code of Ethics states should be done, and what the hospital's policy is for handling this type of situation. Situations that may give rise to conflicts in ethical decision making may include abortion rights and caring for AIDS patients. Ethical problems are not easy problems to deal with; there are usually no right or wrong answers, and solutions are not easily found. Ethical decisions may involve intense feelings that promote arguments and other behaviors not based on reason and thought.

It is incumbent upon the new nurse employee to tell the employer of her or his personal values that may conflict with professional ethics and nursing practice as performed in that facility. Ethical problems and legal issues of nursing care are usually very closely related. Once the patient-nurse relationship is established, the nurse is legally responsible to care for that patient. Also, the nurse is ethically committed to continue care for that patient even though personal values may be compromised. Therefore it is urgent that the nurse notify the appropriate personnel of any specific personal values that may affect the type of patients to be cared for. When personal values conflict with the professional role, a resolution can usually be reached that preserves personal values and allows for professional practice. Nurses must keep in mind that during such a conflict, quality health care must not be compromised.

When conflicts between personal values and agency policy do develop, compromise is usually effective when problem-solving techniques are employed. When conflicts arise concerning patient values (euthanasia), the nurse is obligated to discuss the problem with patients and help them think about alternatives.

It is the nurse's legal and ethical responsibility to report a nurse or a physician who is caring for patients while he or she is under the influence of alcohol or drugs.

Helpful guidelines for ethical decision making include the following:

- Know your values.
- Do not allow your values to be compromised.
- Know your professional nursing ethics.
- Do not allow your nursing ethics to be compromised.
- Do not be disappointed if not everyone agrees with your ethical standards
- Do not force your standards or personal values on anyone else.

The step-by-step approach to **ethical decision making** is as follows:

- Obtain the facts related to the problem.
- Identify the ethical components.
- Identify the ethical agents (people involved).
- Identify options.

Values clarification is a process by which people first examine the things they value and then make choices; it facilitates personal decision making. While it does not include telling people what to do, it helps them toward making their own decisions. It allows for exploration and analysis of the problem and the identification of available choices. Value clarification is a step by step process:

- The first step toward gaining awareness of personal values is to list them. Oftentimes, people act thoughtlessly or hastily because they have not examined or identified their own values. By asking patients to think about what is important or unimportant to them helps identify and clarify their values.

- It is important to be aware of the consequences of an act (risk-benefit). Knowing the consequences and alternatives of a specific value-choice enables the client to make an informed value-choice decision. A goal of nursing is to assist people in becoming familiar with their range of alternatives so that they can then take the time to consider them.

- The client must have the opportunity to choose his or her values freely. It is only then that values can be referred to as true values.

- The client should feel comfortable and satisfied with his or her choice of values. Helping clients examine their feelings about their value choices is a nursing action that can be accomplished by sensitively asking open-ended questions.

- When clients sincerely believe in their choice of values, they will affirm their choice and defend them verbally if necessary.

- Since values are deep-rooted commitments, sections should reflect that commitment.

- Deep-rooted values play a part in the internal and external world of the individual. It becomes intrinsic to his or her whole being, and his or her behavior always reflects that value choice. What people value affects and guides all their actions.

DRILL AND PRACTICE QUESTIONS FOR REVIEW

Complete the statements below.

1. _____ are enforceable rules of conduct made by society.

2. _____ are principles of behavior that informally govern individuals in a society.

3. Children begin to develop a _____ at preschool age.

4. Adolescents begin to use _____ reasoning when making ethical decisions.

5. _____ are deep-rooted, in depth, freely chosen convictions.

6. Needs are internal tensions caused by _____.

7. Safety, security, and protection are _____ level needs.

8. The desire for friendship and love is a _____ level need.

9. Ethical problems in nursing practice usually arise when there is a conflict between _____, _____, and _____.

10. List three guidelines that may be helpful when making ethical decisions: _____, _____, and _____.

11. The sequence used for making ethical decisions is as follows: _____, _____, and _____.

12. The steps used for values clairification include these: _____, _____, _____, _____, _____, _____, and _____.

Determine whether the following statements are TRUE or FALSE.

1. Children under three years of age do not have a sense of what is right or wrong.

2. Nurses should expect that patients will adjust to the nurses' standards or value system.

3. Adolescents always list personal values similar to their parents.

4. Middle and older age adults can easily adapt their values to the changing environment.

5. Values are not the same as needs, beliefs, or interests.

6. The need for food, water, and sleep are first-level needs.

7. Beliefs can easily be interchanged with values because they both reflect the concept of free choice.

8. Codes of ethics are legally binding standards that all nurses must follow.

9. Once the patient-nurse relationship has been established, the nurse is legally and ethically committed to continue care until appropriately relieved.

10. Whenever personal values conflict with professional ethics, nursing students must be prepared to compromise their own personal values.

11. Ethical decisions are easy to make since there is either a right or wrong answer to all problems.

12. Values clarification enables individuals to examine and determine the things they value most.

13. When helping others with values clarification, the nurse should let them know his or her personal values and beliefs.

Situations

Situation 1

As a staff nurse working on a medical unit, you have been assigned to care for Mr. Brown, an eighty-year-old, terminally ill patient. His family disagrees as to whether to continue with life-saving techniques; each family member seems confused as to what to do. As the nurse responsible for Mr. Brown's care, discuss the ethical decision-making guidelines that may be utilized in order to help the family come to a decision. Discuss the nurse's role in this situation.

Situation 2

As a part-time staff nurse, you have been asked to work on a unit where abortions are performed. Because you do not believe in abortions, you do not want to work on that unit. Discuss both the conflicts involved and the responsibilities of the nurse.

ANSWERS TO DRILL AND PRACTICE QUESTIONS

Completion Exercises

1. laws

2. ethics

3. conscience

4. adult

5. values

6. change in the individual or in his or her environment

7. second level

8. third level

9. what the nurse believes, the profession's Code of Ethics, and the agency policy

10. know your own values, know your professional ethics, do not allow your own nursing ethics to be compromised, do not force your personal values on others, do not be disappointed if not everyone meets your expectations

11. obtain the facts, identify the ethical components, identify the people involved, and identify alternatives or options

12. list values, examine possible consequences of the choice, choose freely, feel satisfied with the choice, affirm the choice, act on the choice, and act with a pattern

True/False Exercises

1. T
2. F
3. F
4. F
5. T
6. T
7. F
8. F
9. T
10. F
11. T
12. T
13. F

Situations

Situation 1

First the family members need to have as much information as possible concerning the patient. Second, they need to identify their own feelings about the patient, his life, and his possible death. Third, the family members need to identify possible options to the present course of treatment and the consequences of each option. In addition, the nurse needs to support all the family members during this time and abide by her professional code of ethics and hospital policy for this situation.

Situation 2

Three conflicts may be present in this situation. First, the nurse and the patient may differ in values pertaining to abortion. Second, there may be a conflict between the nurse's own value system and the profession's code of ethics; and third, there may be a conflict between the nurse's personal values and the hospital's policy for this situation. As an individual, the nurse is entitled to a personal value system. It is the nurse's responsibility, however, to share those values pertaining to nursing care with the employer at the initial time of employment. If the employer is unaware of the nurse's personal values, the nurse will be expected to fulfill the obligations of employment listed on the job description. As a professional, the nurse is also expected to render appropriate care within the guidelines of the association's code of ethics. Standard 1 of the ANA's Code of Ethics states, "The nurse provides services with respect for human dignity and the uniqueness of the client unrestricted by considerations of social or economic status, personal attributes, or the nature of health problems." Since the nurse-patient relationship has not begun, the nurse may request that another nurse be assigned to that unit. If the job description clearly indicates that the nurse must care for all types of health problems, the nurse is required to provide such care or seek employment elsewhere.

Chapter 6

NURSING THEORIES

MAJOR NURSING CONCEPTS

A **theory** is a set of interrelated ideas structured in such a way as to explain or predict phenomena. Different **nursing theories** present differing views of nursing. The end result of every nursing theory is to provide the highest level of nursing care possible. Additional goals in the effort by nurse leaders to define a theoretical foundation for nursing practice is to help nurses fully understand, be able to explain, and know why and how they are performing the basic principles of nursing. Knowledge of a specific nursing theory can guide one's nursing care.

Three subjects commonly defined by nursing theorists are **the person to be nursed, the goals of nursing care,** and **the activities of nursing care.**

Several nursing theorists have presented their unique views of nursing. No one theory appears superior to the others, and these different theories tend to be **complementary,** not **contradictory.**

Nursing's first theorist was Florence Nightingale. This theory stresses the physical aspects of nursing care and is referred to as an **environmental theory.** Florence Nightingale believed healing occurs when the nurse changes the client's environment in order to put the client in the best possible condition conducive to health.

Faye Abdellah's theoretical perspective on nursing was defined by listing twenty-one areas of client care thought to encompass the scope of nursing. See pages 00 to 00 in the text. Abdellah's client care list is considered limited; however, it did lay the foundation for other theorists to follow. An important aspect of nursing care—client input—was not stressed by Abdellah.

Hildegard Peplau introduced two important aspects to nursing theory. In addition to physical concerns, Dr. Peplau was concerned with interpersonal relationships. She also advocated nursing plans mutually agreed on by nurse and client. Dr. Peplau's theory is organized using four separate phases of care. During the orientation phase, the nurse helps the client identify and clarify the problem. The client and nurse work together to solve the problem during the identification phase. In the exploitation phase the problem is solved. The therapeutic nurse-client relationship is terminated during the resolution phase.

The integration of basic mental health principles into nursing care was stressed by **Ida Jean Orlando.** This theory includes client input, the dynamic nature of the nurse-client relationship, and the necessity for clients to recognize a need for care that they cannot meet by themselves. The inclusion of client input marks Orlando's theory as innovative for its time in 1968.

Virginia Henderson first defined nursing and then constructed fourteen components of nursing on which care should be devised. Because this theory lacks many specifics that are found in later theories, it is considered incomplete.

Like Peplau, **Dorothea Johnson** emphasized psychological aspects of client care. Because Dr. Johnson's theory integrated physical and psychological client care, nursing theory continued to develop as a holistic concern. Dorothea Johnson developed **seven categories of behavior** to be used as a framework for nursing: security-seeking behavior; nurturance-seeking behavior; mastery of oneself and one's environment; taking in nourishment; ridding the body of wastes; sexual and role identity behavior; and self-protective behavior. Nursing care, according to this theory, is aimed at **reducing client stress** so that the client can better recover from illness.

Another holistic, yet more complex, approach to nursing theory was developed by **Dr. Martha Rogers.** Components of Dr. Rogers' theory closely resemble Systems theory as defined by Bertalanfly. Both uphold the belief that people are more than the sum of their parts and interact continually with their environment. Dr. Rogers also believes that people always have forward momentum, which means they can never go back to what they were before. However, earlier lifetime experiences become part of a person's present state.

Dorothea Orem's self-care theory categorizes nursing into three systems: **wholly compensatory** (a nurse almost totally cares for a client); **partly compensatory** (assists client with self-care); and **supportive-educative** (educates client in those things necessary for self-care).

Imogene King is another nurse theorist who advocates client input into their own nursing care. Her theory includes three assumptions about people: people are **reacting, time oriented,** and **social in nature;** and seven characteristics of people: the abilities **to perceive, to think, to feel, to choose, to set goals, to select means to achieve goals,** and **to make decisions.** In addition, Imogene King describes six processes present during nurse-client interaction: **perception, judgment, action, reaction, interaction,** and **transaction.**

Myra Levine's conservation theory includes four principles of conservation (**conservation of energy, conservation of structural integrity, conservation of personal integrity,** and **conservation of social integrity**) which are present during health and absent in illness. Dr. Levine believes the goal of nursing care is to keep these four elements in proper balance. Interestingly, Levine's physiologic and safety needs and the personal and social elements correlate respectively with Abraham **Maslow's** love needs and self-esteem needs.

Sister Callista Roy's model is termed an **adaption model** because she believes that people cope with environmental changes through adaptive mechanisms. According to this model, people respond to changes by using one or more distinct modes of adapting: **physiological** (the heart beats faster); **self-concept** (the person changes her or his goal to a lesser one); **role function** (the person assumes a passive client role); and **interdependence** (the person relies on others for help). When autonomic nervous system adjustments are made, Sister Roy terms this a **regulator mechanism.** The term **cognator mechanism** refers to thought processes used for adaptation.

DRILL AND PRACTICE QUESTIONS FOR REVIEW

Complete the statements below.

1. The first nursing theory was presented by _____.

2. Florence Nightingale's nursing theory advocated changing the client's _____ in order to support healing.

3. Three areas of nursing usually defined in a nursing theory are _____, _____, and _____.

4. Health care problems are solved during the _____ phase, according to Dr. Peplau's theory.

5. The resolution phase of Dr. Peplau's theory marks the _____ of the nurse-client relationship.

6. The necessity for clients to recognize a need for care that they themselves cannot meet is an important element of _____ nursing theory.

7. The nursing theory commonly referred to as a self-care theory was introduced by _____.

8. In general terms, the goal of nursing according to Dorothea Johnson's nursing theory is to reduce client _____.

9. The nursing theory supporting the notion that people are more than the sum of their parts was developed by _____.

10. The three major categories of nursing care comprising Dorothea Orem's theory are _____, _____, and _____.

11. A nursing theorist whose views are similar to Abraham Maslow's is _____.

12. _____, _____, _____, and _____ are the conservation principles described by Myra Levine.

13. Sister Callista Roy refers to autonomic nervous system adjustments as _____ and adaptive thought processes as _____.

Determine whether the following statements are TRUE or FALSE

1. A nurse cannot use more than one theory to guide her or his practice.

2. An important omission in Abdellah's theory was client-input.

3. Florence Nightingale stressed the psychological aspects of nursing care.

4. According to Faye Abdellah, the nurse makes health care decisions for his or her client.

5. According to Hildegard Peplau, the nurse makes health care decisions in consultation with the client.

6. During the identification phase of Dr. Peplau's theory, the nurse helps the client to identify and clarify the problem.

7. Ida Jean Orlando was the first nurse theorist to emphasize the importance of client-input in one's nursing care.

8. Virginia Henderson's theory of nursing comprises 21 areas of client care.

9. Dorothea Johnson's theory integrated physical and psychological care.

10. Stress reduction in several areas of behavior is a hallmark of Dorothea Johnson's nursing theory.

11. According to Martha Rogers, earlier lifetime experiences have no use in one's present interaction with the environment.

12. Martha Rogers' theory has similarities to Systems theory.

13. Teaching a new mother how to safely bathe her infant would fit into the "partly compensatory" category of Dorothea Orem's theory.

14. An example of a conservation theory is Sister Callista Roy's model.

Identify Orem's Nursing Care System

Identify which type of nursing care according to Dorothea Orem's systems (wholly compensatory, partly compensatory, supportive-educative) the following situations represent.

1. The nurse is caring for a client the day after gall bladder surgery.

2. The nurse is caring for a comatose client.

3. The nurse is discussing different types of birth control with a couple at a Planned Parenthood clinic.

4. The nurse is teaching crutch-walking to an adolescent with a broken ankle.

5. The nurse is helping a client who has suffered a stroke to complete his daily grooming and hygiene.

6. The nurse is caring for a premature infant in the neonatal intensive care unit.

ANSWERS TO DRILL AND PRACTICE QUESTIONS

Completion Exercises

1. Florence Nightingale

2. environment

3. the person to be nursed, the goals of nursing care, and the activities of nursing care

4. exploitation

5. end/termination

6. Ida Jean Orlando's

7. Dorothea Orem

8. stress

9. Martha Rogers

10. wholly compensatory, partly compensatory, and supportive-educative

11. Myra Levine

12. Conservation of energy, conservation of structural integrity, conservation of personal integrity, and conservation of social integrity

13. regulatory mechanisms cognator mechanisms

True/False Exercises

1.	F	8.	F
2.	T	9.	T
3.	F	10.	T
4.	T	11.	F
5.	T	12.	T
6.	F	13.	F
7.	T	14.	F

Identify Orem's Nursing Care System

1. partly compensatory

2. wholly compensatory

3. supportive-educative

4. supportive-educative

5. partly compensatory

6. wholly compensatory

Chapter 7

NURSING RESEARCH AND NURSING PRACTICE

NOTE TO STUDENT

Take special note of the methods of data collection presented in the text in Table 7–2.

MAJOR NURSING CONCEPTS

Research is a systematic process of scientific inquiry aimed at answering questions that need to be answered. As professionals, nurses should participate in the research process so that the quality of patient care can be improved. Participation may be as a **subject**—an actual participant in a research study—or as a **research assistant,** involved in the collection of research data from subjects. All nurses should be skeptical about traditional modes of nursing care and **identify potential researchable problems** for study. Likewise, all nurses must **advocate for patients** to insure that human rights guidelines that direct the conduct of research are adhered to. Subjects in a research study are entitled to privacy, dignity, anonymity, freedom from injury, and informed consent.

Nurses prepared at the baccalaureate level are educated in the reading and **critiquing** of research (reviewing a report of research to determine whether the research process was done appropriately). Only if research studies are read by nurses with some knowledge of the research process can valid research findings that have applicability for nursing practice be appropriately identified. Nurses prepared at the master's and doctoral levels are prepared to conduct research.

There are many different kinds of research studies. **Basic research** is research aimed at generating or testing theories. **Applied research** is research that investigates the application of previously generated theory. **Clinical research** involves examination of specific questions related to the actual implementation of nursing practice. In **experimental research** (empirical research), the researcher attempts to **explain** some factor (dependent variable) by manipulating some other factor (independent variable) that may have an effect on the factor being explained. In **nonexperimental research,** a researcher **describes** the occurrence of some factor(s) or **explores** whether there are associations between certain factors (variables). **Historical research** involves the study and interpretation of past events in order to explain present-day phenomena. **Longitudinal research** involves the collection of data at selected time intervals. **Ex post facto research** involves investigation of something that has already occurred. When the factors being investigated in a research study are quantified (counted), the research is called **quantitative research.** When the factors being studied are simply described and not quantified, the research is called **qualitative research.**

A **research report** begins with an introduction into the researcher's area of interest. A **review of the literature** (which utilizes **primary sources** as well as **secondary sources**) then provides a logical review of prior studies that suggests the need for the researcher's current investigation. The specific **research question** addressed in the research is then stated.

29

In all research studies, some factor, or **variable,** is studied by the researcher. In a research study, there may be a **study variable** (variable described by the researcher), an **independent variable** (factor that has an effect on a dependent variable), a **dependent variable** (factor affected by an independent variable), and/or **extraneous (intervening) variables** (factors other than an independent variable that affect the dependent variable). Every effort must be made by the researcher to control for the effect of extraneous variables on the variable of interest to the researcher. In experimental or nonexperimental studies in which a researcher investigates an association between variables, the researcher may make a statement regarding the results he or she expects to find. This statement is called a **hypothesis.**

The research **methodology** includes the specific design (plan) used to answer the research questions, setting (location), sampling technique, and data collection procedures. A **research design** is the researcher's plan for answering the research question—the design can be experimental or nonexperimental. New areas of research are most appropriately studied using a nonexperimental design. Areas that have been previously studied can be further studied with the use of experimental designs. Regardless of the research design, the **setting** chosen by the researcher as the location for the study should be appropriate to the answering of the research question.

The group of subjects from which data are collected in a research study is called a **sample.** This group is a subset of a larger group, called a **sample population,** to which the researcher would like to **generalize** findings obtained from the sample. In order to generalize findings obtained from a sample, however, the researcher should try to obtain a sample that is **representative of** (similar to) the sample population. With the use of a **random (probability) sampling** technique, each person in the sample population has an equal chance of being chosen as a subject in the sample, and the researcher is assured that the sample is representative of the sample population. Random samples are preferred over **convenience (nonprobability) samples.** Besides random sampling, the use of large samples also helps to insure that a sample is representative of the sample population. In descriptive studies, the sample should be 10 to 20 percent of persons from the sample population. In studies investigating associations, the sample should include a minimum of 20 to 30 subjects for each group studied.

Data in a research study can be collected by observation, physiological measurement, personal interview, or questionnaire. Regardless of the method used, the researcher must insure that the method has **validity** (measures what it is supposed to measure) and **reliability** (consistently obtains the same results). In a research report, the researcher should discuss the means by which validity and reliability were determined. A reported reliability of .8 or above is very good. When more than one observer is used, the means by which the researcher insured that each observer observed in a similar fashion should be addressed **(interrater reliability).**

The actual data obtained from subjects in a research study are called **raw data.** In a qualitative research study, raw data are analyzed by **content analysis,** in which the data are reviewed to identify themes. In a quantitative study, data are quantified with the use of statistics.

Regardless of the type of research study, **descriptive statistics** are used to summarize the characteristics of the sample. **Frequencies** (the number of times a certain value on a variable occurred in the sample) are usually reported. **Measures of central tendency,** single numbers that represent the middle of the sample group on any one variable, and **measures of variability,** numbers that describe how much dispersion there was in a sample on any one variable, are also usually reported. Measures of central tendency include the **mean** (average score), the **median** (middle score), and the **mode** (most frequently occurring score). Measures of variability include the **range** (span between the highest and lowest values on any one variable) and the **standard deviation** (average deviation of all scores from the mean score).

Other types of statistics computed in research studies include correlation statistics, the Chi-Square test, the t-test, and Analysis of Variance. A **correlation** can range from -1.0 to +1.0. The number and the sign reflect whether or not there is a relationship between two variables. The higher the number, the stronger association there is between the two variables (they vary together). The sign reflects the direction of the association (the association between the two variables can be in the same [+] or opposite [-] direction). When a researcher needs to determine if there are differences between groups on certain variables, the **Chi-Square test,** the **t-test,** or the **Analysis of Variance** is used.

As a result of data analysis and the computation of statistics in many research studies, researchers report whether or not their hypothesis (expected association) was supported at a specific level of significance. When a researcher reports a level of significance, **inferential statistics** have been utilized, and the results of the study can be generalized from the sample to the sample population (assuming a representative sample). The **level of significance,** also called the p value or alpha (α) value, reflects the likelihood that the association found by the researcher was due to chance (how much risk the researcher was willing to take that his or her findings are not true). It is important for nurses reading research reports to determine whether or not the researcher used an appropriate level of significance for testing the research hypothesis in the particular study reported. A commonly used and usually appropriate level of significance in nursing research studies is .05 (researcher willing to be wrong 5 in 100 times).

Once data analysis is complete, a researcher is able to generate conclusions from his or her study. These **conclusions** should be logical and recommend use of findings in practice only when appropriate.

DRILL AND PRACTICE QUESTIONS FOR REVIEW

Complete the statements below.

1. Nurses prepared at the _____ level are minimally qualified to critique the report of a research study.

2. The rights of persons involved in research studies have evolved from initial guidelines provided in the _____.

3. Research conducted by nurse clinicians in association with experienced nurse researchers is called _____ research.

4. A nurse researcher conducts a research study to determine the most effective turning protocol for the prevention of decubitus ulcers. In this study, the independent variable is _____ and the dependent variable is _____.

5. A case study analysis is an example of _____ research.

6. Whenever a researcher manipulates some factor in a study to determine its effect on another factor, the researcher is conducting _____ research.

7. A researcher conducts a study and collects data from the same subjects every six months for three years. This kind of study is called _____ research.

8. Data from interviews conducted as part of a qualitative study is analyzed by _____.

9. _____ sources are preferred as references in a research report.

10. A researcher is studying the effect of noise on learning. Lighting my also affect learning. The researcher places all subjects in rooms with similar lighting to _____ for the effect of lighting on learning. In this study, lighting is a/an _____ variable.

11. A researcher investigates which nursing intervention is most effective in teaching self-administration of a medication. Four different interventions are tried with four similar groups of patients. The sample size should be _____.

12. A nurse researcher develops a questionnaire aimed at determining what people know about organ donation. Before using the questionnaire, it is shown to experts in the field of organ donation. Their comments are used to revise the questionnaire to make it more appropriate. With this process, the researcher is attempting to make the questionnaire _____.

Determine whether the following statements are TRUE or FALSE.

1. The primary purpose of nursing research is to establish nursing as a profession.

2. Potential research subjects should not be told about the possible risks involved in being a research subject, because this information may discourage participation.

3. All research studies should have a hypothesis.

4. Convenience sampling is preferred over random sampling.

5. It would be appropriate for a researcher to utilize and make recommendations from use of a test for which an internal consistency reliability of .25 was obtained.

6. A correlation of +.7 between age and scores on a math test indicates that as age increases, scores on the math test also increase.

7. If a researcher reports that his or her findings were significant at the .10 level of significance, it means that he or she was willing to be wrong 1 in 100 times.

For each of the following research problems, state whether the italicized words refer to the independent variable or the dependent variable in the study.

1. Is there a relationship between *educational preparation of the nurse* and nurse effectiveness?

2. Is there a difference in *postop anxiety* of patients based on type of preop teaching received?

3. Does quantity of fluid consumed in the diet affect *number of bowel movements?*

4. Does *education level* affect ability to read newspaper articles?

5. Does the death of a spouse affect *self-esteem?*

Match the statistic in column A with its appropriate use from column B.

Column A	Column B
1. mean	a. average deviation of each subject's score from the mean score
2. median	b. most frequently occurring score
3. mode	c. middle score
4. range	d. average score
5. standard deviation	e. spread of scores

ANSWERS TO DRILL AND PRACTICE QUESTIONS

Completion Exercises

1. baccalaureate
2. Nuremberg Articles
3. collaborative
4. turning protocol, prevention of decubitus ulcers
5. nonexperimental or descriptive
6. experimental
7. longitudinal
8. content analysis
9. primary
10. control; extraneous or intervening
11. 8–120
12. valid

True/False Exercises

1. F
2. F
3. F
4. F
5. F
6. T
7. F

Determine the Variable

1. independent variable
2. dependent variable
3. dependent variable
4. independent variable
5. dependent variable

Matching

1. d
2. c
3. b
4. e
5. a

Chapter 8

LEADERSHIP IN NURSING

NOTE TO STUDENT

Take special note of text Table 8-2, Basic Principles of Leadership.

MAJOR NURSING CONCEPTS

Leadership is the ability to influence others in order to reach a specific goal. Nurses need to be leaders because they coordinate patient care and manage the activities of other health care professionals. Effective leaders have the ability to communicate clearly, are knowledgeable role models, demonstrate respect for others, and are fair and flexible. Empathy, motivational skills, and trustworthiness are additional characteristics necessary in leaders who help people adjust to change.

Leaders are frequently called upon to introduce new and different ideas. **Change** is complex, often beneficial, energy expending, and prone to resistance. Initiating change is often difficult. **Steward (1959)** has described **identification, reassurance, communication, participation, mutual interest,** and **follow-through** as the six important steps for initiating change.

Nurses often initiate change in individuals and in **groups.** Common types of groups are occupational, social, educational, recreational, or health related. **Group content** is the set of topics discussed in a group while **group process** is the verbal and nonverbal communications occurring within the group. To be an effective group leader, a nurse must understand and be able to influence both content and process.

An **advocate** is a leader who acts to improve existing conditions on behalf of another person. The nurse advocate may assist people in making decisions about their health care or in obtaining appropriate health care services for a client in a complex bureaucratic system. Successful advocates follow lines of authority, are resourceful, objective, and able to solve problems.

Assertiveness refers to the ability to communicate your feeling without violating others' feelings or rights. Assertiveness is a necessary characteristic for leadership. Providing the best-quality nursing care possible and acting as patient advocate often require assertive behavior on the part of the nurse.

The process of building professional associations to obtain information, influence, or power is called **networking,** which enhances the nurse's competence as an advocate and leader.

Nurse leaders utilize different methods for delivering nursing care to clients. Using the **case method,** the nurse is assigned the full care of each patient assigned to her or him. **Functional nursing** is often referred to as an "assembly-line" method because each nurse does the same small portion of care for all patients. **Team nursing** requires a skilled registered nurse who leads a team of various nursing personnel. This team is then responsible for the total care of a number of clients. the **primary nursing** care system requires the nurse to plan and direct the total care of a client twenty-four hours a day, utilizing associate nurses for the hours when the primary nurse is unavailable.

DRILL AND PRACTICE QUESTIONS FOR REVIEW

Complete the statements below.

1. The leadership style most effective in an emergency is _____.
2. According to Steward (1959), the six steps important for initiating changes are _____, _____, _____, _____, _____, and _____.
3. Two elements of group dynamics are group _____ and _____.
4. The use of fraudulent treatments is called _____.
5. The agency concerned with food and drug safety in the United States is _____.
6. When a person is able to make her or his feelings known without infringing on others' feelings, this person is exhibiting _____ behavior.
7. An emergency room nurse consulting with a psychiatric nurse specialist is an example of _____.
8. Name three different levels of nursing personnel:

   _____

   _____

   _____

9. Name four different nursing care delivery methods:

   _____

   _____

   _____

   _____

10. The nursing organizational method used most often today is _____.

Determine whether the following statements are TRUE or FALSE.

1. Leadership and authority are synonymous.
2. One method a nurse may use to decrease resistance to change is to encourage the individuals affected by the change to participate in planning change.
3. Adjustment to change is easier when change is immediate and rapid.
4. Effective advocacy requires organized planning and action.
5. Anger is a useful tool for the nurse advocate.
6. Assertiveness and aggression are synonymous.
7. Assertive behavior requires energy.
8. Head nurses or patient care coordinators are responsible for the quality of nursing care on their particular unit twenty-four hours a day.

9. Today private duty nurses practice the case method of nursing care.

10. People who request second opinions are unusually anxious and distrustful.

Identify the Leadership Style

Identify the leadership style (autocratic, laissez-faire, democratic) in each of the following situations.

1. The nurse teaches a patient with high blood pressure the importance of a low salt diet.

2. A nurse in an intensive care unit tells a nurse's aide to bring the emergency cart to room 102 immediately.

3. A nurse discusses with a breast cancer patient the different surgical choices offered by the patient's surgeon.

4. A nurse in the emergency room wraps one-year-old Bobby in a restraining "papoose" in order to start a necessary intravenous infusion.

5. The head nurse of the pediatric unit requests proposals for a new work schedule for and from the staff.

Situations

Situation 1

The head nurse of a medical-surgical unit wants to institute a new method for the administration of medications. Describe how the nurse could reach this goal using the autocratic, laissez-faire, and democratic leadership styles.

Situation 2

Mrs. Jones is a seventy-five-year -old woman who is hospitalized for a fractured hip. The fracture was surgically repaired, and the nurse is planning Mrs. Jones's discharge. Mrs. Jones has voiced several concerns: "I can't swallow these big pills"; "I'll never be able to get in and out of my bed"; "I live alone"; "Being sick is very expensive." Relevant to the advocacy role of the nurse, what suggestions would you include in your nursing care plan?

ANSWERS TO DRILL AND PRACTICE QUESTIONS

Completion Exercises

1. autocratic
2. identification, reassurance, communication, participation, mutual interest, follow-through
3. content and process
4. quackery
5. The Federal Food and Drug Administration
6. assertive
7. networking
8. registered nurse

    licensed practical nurse

    nurse's aide
9. case

    functional

    team

    primary
10. primary nursing

True/False Exercises

1. F
2. T
3. F
4. T
5. F
6. F
7. T
8. T
9. T
10. F

Identify the Leadership Style

1. democratic
2. autocratic
3. laissez-faire
4. autocratic
5. democratic

Situations

Situation 1

1. *Autocratic:* Simply inform the staff of the new policy and institute this policy.

2. *Laissez-faire:* Allow each nurse to try independently his or her own method.

3. *Democratic:* Encourage the nurses to propose and discuss several possible methods and allow the nurses to vote on one method.

Situation 2

- Request from the pharmacy a liquid form of Mrs. Jones's medication.
- Discuss with her family the possibility of renting a hospital bed for Mrs. Jones's use at home.
- Notify Mrs. Jones's local church group of her need for visitors and companionship.
- Discuss Mrs. Jones's post-discharge nursing care needs with the physician and the community health nurses.
- Determine whether Mrs. Jones is eligible for nonmedical services such as "Meals-on Wheels."
- Arrange for a social worker to visit Mrs. Jones to discuss available financial aid.

PART III

THE NURSING PROCESS

Chapter 9

NURSING PROCESS: ASSESSMENT

MAJOR NURSING CONCEPTS

The **nursing process** is the framework in which nurses provide client care. It is a series of steps that include the collection of data about a client (**assessment**), the understanding of that data (**analysis**), the determination of client problems (**nursing diagnosis**), the **planning and implementation** of care, and the **evaluation** of care provided. Nurses use the nursing process to problem solve, make decisions about client care on an ongoing basis, and to plan care comprehensively in the form of **nursing care plans.**

In the **assessment** phase, the nurse establishes a pertinent and individualized data base of relevant client information. This data base is complete (total history and physical data, etc.) if the nurse must plan comprehensive care; it is selective if the nurse has identified specific client problems for which care is to be planned. The data base of information is obtained from a client's health history (determined by interview), physical examination, and auxiliary data, such as laboratory and X-ray results.

Data collected as part of assessment is categorized as **subjective** (a symptom reported by the client) or **objective** (a sign observed by the nurse). When obtained data deviate from normal, they are called **positive findings;** normal or healthy data are termed **negative findings.** Data that a nurse obtains directly from a client are called **primary source data;** that obtained from sources other than the client are termed **secondary source data.** Both **disabilities** (characteristics detrimental to high-level wellness) and **abilities** (activities or functions a person does well) are data to collect as part of assessment. In the collection of all types of client data, the nurse should assume a neutral, objective, and unbiased approach, and then attempt to confirm or verify the accuracy of the data.

Health interviewing involves the gathering of client data through a systematic question-and-answer process and simultaneous observation of the client's facial expressions and body language. The setting for the interview should be conducive to the expression of feelings and factual information (private, quiet, comfortable setting). Clients should be advised regarding the name and role of the nurse conducting the interview and the specific reason(s) for the interview. Fact-finding and open-ended questions, in conjunction with transition statements and supportive comments (which reassure clients that they can discuss anything they wish) are most effective in obtaining necessary data. Vague, critical, compound, leading, and sophisticated questions should be avoided.

A **physical examination** should also be conducted in a systematic fashion. The techniques of **inspection** (looking), **palpation** (touching), **percussion** (checking the density of body parts), and **auscultation** (listening) are utilized. Nurses are responsible for continued assessments that reflect total body function, although their examinations often focus on assessments pertinent to particular health problems that a client experiences.

Auxiliary data that supplement health history and physical examination data include the reports of lab tests, X-rays, and consultations.

Once data have been collected, categorization of the data into a framework (such as Gordon's functional health patterns) can help to insure that data collection is complete.

DRILL AND PRACTICE QUESTIONS FOR REVIEW

Complete the statements below.

1. The five steps of the nursing process include these: _____, _____, _____, _____, and _____.

2. A nurse identifies a client problem that can be solved by nurses. The nursing process term for this problem is _____.

3. In the evaluation phase of the nursing process, the nurse determines if _____ have been achieved.

4. Assessment information is obtained from a client's _____, _____, and _____.

5. When interviewing a client, a nurse explains what is coming next in the interview. This statement is called a _____ statement.

6. In collecting health history data, a nurse determines that a client's weight is not normal for his height and weight. This is a _____ finding.

Determine whether the following statements are TRUE or FALSE.

1. When obtaining a health history on a child, a large part of the history revolves around the mother's pregnancy.

2. When interviewing clients, the nurse should remain standing so that a professional atmosphere is maintained.

3. To make people feel comfortable during an interview, the use of first names if preferred.

4. When interviewing clients, it is appropriate to criticize clients about behaviors that are not health-producing.

5. A nurse is using the assessment skill of auscultation when he or she listens for sounds as a finger is used to check the density of a body part.

For each of the data listed below, state the functional health pattern category into which it would fall, according to Gordon's typology.

1. number of bowel movements a client has per day

2. type of exercise performed by a client each day

3. number of hours of sleep a client has each night

4. amount of fluid a client drinks daily

5. what client does when he or she is ill

6. client's comfort level

7. client's ability to conceive children

8. client's feelings about his or her body

State whether each of the following would be appropriately classified as subjective or objective data.

1. client's description of his or her pain

2. client's red blood cell count

3. client's skin color as observed by the nurse

4. client's blood pressure as determined by the nurse

5. color of client's urine as observed by the nurse

ANSWERS TO DRILL AND PRACTICE QUESTIONS

Completion Exercises

1. assessment, analysis, planning, implementation, evaluation

2. nursing diagnosis

3. goals

4. health history, physical examination, auxiliary data

5. transition

6. positive

True/False Exercises

1. T
2. F

3. F
4. F
5. F

State the Pattern

1. elimination pattern

2. activity-exercise pattern

3. sleep-rest pattern

4. nutritional-metabolic pattern

5. health-perception/health-management pattern

6. self-perception/self-concept pattern

7. sexuality-reproductive pattern

8. self-perception/self-concept pattern

State the Type of Data

1. subjective
2. objective
3. objective
4. objective
5. objective

Chapter 10

NURSING PROCESS: ANALYSIS AND NURSING DIAGNOSIS

NOTE TO STUDENT

Pay special attention to Table 10-6 and the box in this chapter that provide guidance in the identification and writing of nursing diagnoses.

MAJOR NURSING CONCEPTS

In the **analysis** phase of the nursing process, the nurse studies and interprets data to determine a client's health care needs (**nursing diagnoses**).

A client's health care needs are determined from the perspective of his or her concept of optimal health (e.g., self-care ability, adaptation ability, functional ability of all body systems). Client needs may also be determined using **Maslow's Hierarchy of Needs.** According to Maslow, a **need** is an unmet desire, and a person will strive to have unmet desires fulfilled in a priority fashion, (physiological, safety and security, love and belonging, self-esteem, self-actualization needs).

The organization of data into categories facilitates their examination to determine if data collection has been complete. Furthermore, abnormal and pertinent normal findings can easily be identified and interpreted so that problems can be identified.

A **nursing diagnosis** is a problem (unmet need) that a nurse can treat. It is an **actual** or **potential** response to a physiological or psychological health problem. It should be stated in PES format (problem, etiology, signs and symptoms or defining characteristics). The **etiology** of a client's problem refers to the factor causing the problem. When included in the nursing diagnostic statement, it is connected to the nursing problem with the words "related to." **Signs and symptoms** are objective and/or subjective data that substantiate a client's problem. Nursing diagnoses should be clear, specific, and utilize NANDA (North American Nursing Association of Nursing Diagnoses) terminology, whenever possible.

A client's nursing diagnoses should be dealt with in priority fashion. Problems that are life-threatening and/or pose a threat to something highly valued by a client take greatest priority. Maslow's hierarchy can also be used to determine priority nursing diagnoses.

DRILL AND PRACTICE QUESTIONS FOR REVIEW

Complete the statements below.

1. The analysis phase of the nursing process includes: _____.

2. According to Maslow, activity is classified as a _____ need.

3. An individual feels a sense of personal growth and maturity and fully satisfied with life. This individual would be classified, according to Maslow, as _____.

4. A nursing diagnostic statement should include three parts: _____, _____, and _____.

5. When writing a nursing diagnosis, the words _____ should be used to connect the statement of a client's problem to the etiology.

6. When prioritizing nursing diagnoses, the nurse should consider: _____, _____, _____, _____, and _____.

Determine whether the following statements are TRUE or FALSE.

1. During the analysis phase of the nursing process, only positive findings from a client's data base are examined.

2. Medical diagnoses are useful in determining nursing diagnoses.

3. The use of NANDA diagnoses helps to standardize nursing terminology.

4. Only NANDA diagnoses are acceptable when stating nursing diagnoses.

5. Nursing diagnoses should be prioritized.

6. It is preferable for clients and support persons to be involved in identification of nursing problems.

Using Maslow's hierarchy, place the following needs in priority order.

sleep

personal growth

freedom from pain

independence

cleanliness

dignity

oxygen

State why each of the following nursing diagnostic statements is incorrect.

1. Pain due to surgery as noted by facial grimace.

2. Asthma related to strawberry allergy as noted by difficulty in breathing.

3. Alteration in comfort.

4. Anemia due to low hemoglobin level as evidenced by fatigue.

ANSWERS TO DRILL AND PRACTICE QUESTIONS

Completion Exercises

1. interpretation of data and determination of nursing diagnoses
2. physiological
3. self-actualized
4. problem, etiology, signs and symptoms or defining characteristics
5. related to
6. the life-threatening nature of the client's problem, how serious the problem is to the client, the cost of resolving the problem, the feasibility of resolving the problem, the time it will take to resolve the problem

True/False Exercises

1. F
2. T
3. T

4. F
5. T
6. T

Place in Priority Order

oxygen

sleep

cleanliness

freedom from pain

independence

dignity

personal growth

Incorrect Nursing Diagnoses

1. Instead of the word *pain*, the NANDA statement, "Alteration in comfort," would be more appropriate; the words *due to* should be replaced with *related to*.
2. Asthma is a medical diagnosis, not a nursing diagnosis.
3. Etiology and signs and symptoms are missing.
4. Enemia is a medical diagnosis, not a nursing diagnosis; the words *due to* should be replaced with *related to*.

Chapter 11

NURSING PROCESS: PLANNING AND IMPLEMENTATION

NOTE TO STUDENT

Be sure to review the Principles of Planning and Implementation that are highlighted in a Focus section in this chapter. Also, review the nursing care plans that are highlighted in box fashion.

MAJOR NURSING CONCEPTS

The **planning** phase of the nursing process involves the selection of **goals** for care and the determination and statement of strategies or plans for care (**nursing orders**) to achieve goals. Once nursing diagnoses have been identified, goal-setting is accomplished. Goals may relate to helping a client cope with a health problem or keeping the client well. A **goal** or **behavioral objective** is something that is to be achieved by the client (a behavior of the client). It should be directly related to a problem/nursing diagnosis that has been identified. Clients and support persons should be involved in setting goals for care, as feasible. Goals should be realistic and specifically state what is to be accomplished, in measurable terms. They should include **criteria** by which achievement of the goal will be measured. They should also include a **time frame** that reflects the time in which the goal is to be achieved. **Long-term goals** (more comprehensive) should be determined first. **Short-term goals** lead to achievement of long-term goals. As with nursing diagnoses, goals of care should be prioritized.

Nursing orders should be specific, realistic, stated in consecutive order, and should designate who will be responsible for the care or action prescribed. Often, **collaboration** with other health care providers is appropriate, and nursing orders may designate them as initiators of some aspects of care. Nursing orders may evolve from medical diagnoses or prescriptions but should include only **nursing** actions. Each nursing action planned should have a sound **rationale** (reason why the action should work to achieve the goal).

To insure that all nurses caring for a client are consistent in provision of care and to insure high quality care, one **nursing care plan** (written plan of care) is developed for each client, although all nurses caring for the client should have continuous input in the development and revision of the care plan. Often, written care plans become a permanent part of a client's record. Every nursing care plan should include a client's nursing diagnoses, goals for each nursing diagnosis, and nursing orders for each goal. Rationale for prescribed actions are assumed and not written by practicing nurses; student nurses must include rationale in written care plans. **Standardized care plans** (incorporate general care appropriate for clients with specific medical and/or nursing diagnoses) are efficient and time-saving; however, they must be individualized to be effective.

The **implementation** of care involves the carrying out of planned nursing actions (also called **nursing therapies** or **nursing interventions**). Implementation may involve **health maintenance** (wellness care) or **assisting a client to accept inevitable death.** Health maintenance care includes **primary (health promotion, prevention of illness), secondary (restoration of health), and tertiary (rehabilitation to optimal health) prevention.** Implementation can include the carrying out of actions that are **dependent** (must be prescribed by another health care provider), **interdependent** (actions are determined in collaboration with another health care provider), or **independent** (actions are determined by nurses alone). When administering care, nurses provide direct care, supervise care, coordinate care, make referrals, teach (supply answers or information) clients and support persons, provide anticipatory guidance (a form of teaching, done in anticipation of health problems or questions that may arise), implement psychomotor skills (require integration of thought and motor activity), and counsel (help clients find answers to their questions or problems), comfort, protect, and support clients.

DRILL AND PRACTICE QUESTIONS FOR REVIEW

Complete the statements below.

1. Plans or actions determined by nurses to achieve client care goals are called _____.

2. A nursing care plan that has been developed for use with all clients who have had abdominal surgery is called a _____ care plan.

3. Every nursing care plan written by practicing nurses should include _____, _____, and _____.

4. A nurse advises a client that he should have a yearly dental exam. This is an example of _____ prevention.

5. A nurse administers a client an enema. The nurse must know how to use the equipment properly and understand how the procedure may affect the client. This is an example of a _____ skill.

Determine whether the following statements are TRUE or FALSE.

1. All nursing orders should evolve from medical diagnoses and medical orders.

2. A nurse wishes to perform postop exercises with a client who has had orthopedic surgery. Because of the specific surgery, the nurse cannot initiate exercise with the client until the physician prescribes specific exercises. When the nurse begins to implement exercises with the client, the nurse will be implementing an interdependent nursing action.

3. When the nurse teaches a client who recently had a left leg amputation about the use of a prosthesis, the nurse is carrying out tertiary prevention.

4. When a nurse collaborates with other health care providers to arrange for a meeting regarding the care of a client, the nurse is assuming the role of supervisor.

5. Counseling a client involves advising him or her what the best approach in a situation would be.

State why each of the nursing orders listed below is incorrect.

1. Turn client frequently.

2. Client will ambulate three times a day.

3. Make sure client eats.

4. Teach support persons procedure for dressing change.

5. Administer prescribed meds.

State why each of the following goal statements is incorrect.

1. Mrs. Jones will understand her diet.
2. Mr. Jackson will ambulate 10 feet.
3. Ms. Smith will be comfortable.

ANSWERS TO DRILL AND PRACTICE QUESTIONS

Completion Exercises

1. nursing orders
2. standardized
3. nursing diagnoses, goals for care, nursing orders
4. primary
5. psychomotor

True/False Exercises

1. F
2. F

3. T
4. F
5. F

Incorrect Statements of Nursing Orders

1. Does not state who is to turn client, exactly how often client should be turned, or in what direction/position client should be turned.
2. Does not state who will ambulate client, when ambulate will be done, or how much ambulation will be accomplished.
3. Does not state who will make sure the client eats, what meals will be monitored, or exactly how much the client is to eat.
4. Does not state who will do the teaching, who the support persons are, where dressing is located, or exactly what is to be taught.
5. Does not state who will administer medications, what the medications are, or when medications are to be administered.

Incorrect Goal Statements

1. the word *understand* is vague and not measurable; a time frame must be stated; criteria for evaluation of goal achievement should be stated
2. a time frame must be stated; criteria for evaluation of goal achievement should be stated
3. the word *comfortable* is vague and not measurable; a time frame must be stated; criteria for evaluation of goal achievement should be stated

Chapter 12

NURSING PROCESS: EVALUATION

NOTE TO STUDENT

Review the examples of nursing process application in an ambulatory and an in-patient setting provided in the chapter. These demonstrate utilization of the entire nursing process in determination and implementation of a nursing care plan.

MAJOR NURSING CONCEPTS

In the **evaluation** phase of the nursing process, the nurse determines if goal criteria have been met. Subjective and objective data are utilized. If criteria have been met, established plans of care are continued. If criteria have not been met, nursing orders and/or implementation of care are modified as necessary. Reassessment of data and a new plan of care may need to be accomplished.

To determine if goal criteria have been met, client input is necessary. In addition, the nurse must determine if implementations have been satisfactory. If goal criteria have not been met, data reassessment should occur to determine if established nursing diagnoses are appropriate. Goals and criteria should be examined to insure that they are realistic and appropriate for the individual client. Nursing orders should be reexamined to determine if they are comprehensive, specific, and realistic. Implementations should be examined to determine if they have consistently been carried out as specified.

Evaluation of care may be accomplished by individual nurses or by a group of health care providers (nurses and/or others). Evaluation may be done informally or formally (with the use of a written checklist, for example). Upon discharge of a client from a health care facility, a general, formal and informal evaluation of care provided and goal achievement should be accomplished. Periodic, formal, comprehensive assessment of the quality of care delivered by caregivers in a health care facility is accomplished through **audit.**

DRILL AND PRACTICE QUESTIONS FOR REVIEW

Complete the statements below.

1. _____ and _____ data are examined in the evaluation phase of the nursing process to determine if goal criteria have been met.

2. For accreditation purposes, health care agencies periodically evaluate the quality of care provided by the nursing staff. This evaluation process is called _____.

3. Achievement of _____ is determined in the evaluation phase of the nursing process.

4. When a nurse determines that planned nursing actions have not consistently been carried out, the nurse has identified a problem in the _____ phase of the nursing process.

5. When a nurse determines that it is unrealistic to expect a client to be able to ambulate as much as had been anticipated, the nurse has identified a problem in the _____ phase of the nursing process.

Determine whether the following statements are TRUE or FALSE.

1. All steps of the nursing process should be reexamined in the evaluation phase of the nursing process.

2. Evaluation is best accomplished by the individual nurse responsible for the development of a client's care plan.

3. When formal evaluation checklists are developed, outcome measures should be vague enough to allow for subjectivity on the part of the evaluator.

4. Evaluation of client progress is an important part of a discharge summary.

5. It is unlikely that nursing diagnoses established for a client at the beginning of a hospital stay will vary as the client approaches discharge.

ANSWERS TO DRILL AND PRACTICE QUESTIONS

Completion Exercises

1. subjective, objective
2. audit
3. goals
4. implementation
5. planning

True/False Exercises

1.	T	3.	F
2.	F	4.	T
		5.	F

PART IV

HEALTH AS A DYNAMIC FORCE

Chapter 13

HEALTH AND ILLNESS

NOTE TO STUDENT

Review Table 13-1, which summarizes wellness/illness behaviors.

MAJOR NURSING CONCEPTS

Health is a concept that has been defined in various ways. According to the **World Health Organization,** healthy individuals are free of physical symptoms of disease and feel good about their present state. A more recent definition describes health as an illusion that we strive for throughout life **(Dubos).** Nurse theorists have variously defined health as a dynamic life cycle state **(King),** a state determined by social groups and absence of pathologic conditions **(Levine),** a condition characterized by the ability of the whole person to function **(Orem),** and the process of being integrated and whole **(Roy).** According to **Dunn,** health and illness are inseparable entities that fall on a continuum. In general, health is recognized as a dynamic state that is achieved only if people successfully adapt to changes in their internal and external environments. Nurses help people adapt so that optimal wellness can be achieved. Wellness behaviors reflect activity, self-fulfillment, self-care ability, a preventive approach, independence, and responsibility.

Statistics are used to reflect the incidence of health and illness. Mor**bidity** statistics reflect incidence of disease; **mortality** statistics reflect incidence of death. **Infant mortality** statistics (annual number of deaths of infants less than one year old) reflect a nation's overall health. Mortality statistics enable us to see that heart disease and cancer are the leading causes of death in the United States. **U.S. health goals** reflect a desire to further improve infant health and reduce the infant mortality rate; to improve the health and reduce the mortality rate in children, adolescents, and adults; and to improve the health and quality of life for older adults.

Illness occurs for a variety of reasons (altered defenses, metabolic disease, altered growth, trauma, chromosomal abnormality, nutrient disorders, psychosocial disorders) and depends on individual and/or environmental factors (age, sex, mental status, mental outlook, physiological coping ability, pain threshold, economic status, support systems, culture, seasonal variations, use of safety precautions, and availability and use of prevention services). Illness affects families and communities as well as individuals; nurses are especially necessary in helping people adapt to chronic (long-term) illness.

Health practices meant to keep people healthy vary by age group:

Infancy: prenatal care, routine health examinations and immunizations, proper nutrition, strong parent-child relationship

Childhood: Routine immunizations and participation in health screening programs, good eating habits and normal weight, dental hygiene and care, automobile and recreation safety, enriching experiences for mental and physical growth

Adolescence and Young Adulthood: Safe driving behaviors and safe use of firearms, education regarding the hazards of drugs and cigarette smoking, good nutrition, and effective patterns for relating to others and coping with stress

Middle-aged Adulthood: Periodic health exams, sound nutrition and exercise habits, reduction in smoking/alcohol intake, use of preventive health services, automobile safety, self-examination of breasts or testicles, use of effective mechanisms for coping with stress

Older Adulthood: Maintenance of physical and mental activity and sound nutrition practices, use of health care services and community resources, awareness of the possibility of drug interactions

DRILL AND PRACTICE QUESTIONS FOR REVIEW

Complete the statements below.

1. The _____ rate refers to the incidence of disease; the _____ rate refers to the incidence of death.

2. The point at which an individual feels pain is called his or her _____.

3. A diet rich in saturated fats may prone an individual to the health problem, _____.

4. _____ infections tend to occur more frequently during the winter months.

5. Currently, the life expectancy of a male is _____ years; of a female, _____ years.

6. The most serious threats to infant health include _____ and _____.

7. Low birth weight infants are more frequently born to mothers who _____, _____, _____, _____, _____, or _____.

8. Among adolescents, the incidence of _____ has increased dramatically.

9. Overall, the mortality rate has declined, except among _____.

10. Middle-aged adults should be taught to limit the amount of _____ in their diet to prevent cardiovascular disease.

Determine whether the following statements are TRUE or FALSE.

1. High-level wellness is achieved once an individual is free of all physical illness.

2. The incidence of lung cancer and cardiovascular disease is greater in men than in women.

3. In general, older adults should be advised to limit their activity so that their cardiovascular system is not overly stressed.

4. In general, parents of a handicapped child cope better if they are not immediately made aware of a newborn child's handicap.

5. Alleviating stress in a person experiencing pain can also help alleviate pain.

ANSWERS TO DRILL AND PRACTICE QUESTIONS

Completion Exercises

1. morbidity, mortality
2. pain threshold
3. atherosclerosis
4. respiratory
5. 70, 77
6. low birth weight, birth defects
7. are adolescents, have no prenatal care, have poor nutrition, smoke, use alcohol or drugs, have low economic status
8. sexually transmitted diseases
9. adolescents
10. cholesterol

True/False Exercises

1. F
2. T

3. F
4. F
5. T

Chapter 14

HEALTH BELIEFS AND BEHAVIORS

MAJOR NURSING CONCEPTS

Illness affects different people in different ways. For example, people often respond to signs of illness by either seeking help or by delaying asking for help as long as possible.

Rosenstack's health belief model provides a framework for assessing a person's perception of the seriousness of an illness, factors which modify a person's perception of illnesses (knowledge, age, intellectual level, advice from others), and the likelihood of a person seeking help for a health problem (dependent on barriers and benefits).

Parsons's stages of illness include the transition, acceptance, and convalescence stages. The first phase of the **transition stage is** called **symptom awareness** and refers to the recognition of symptoms such as pain, nausea, or dizziness. The second phase of transition is the "confirmation of illness" and is characterized by discussing symptoms with friends and family. As the person realizes he or she needs to seek health care, he or she has entered the stage of acceptance. Once health care is sought, the person adopts **"a sick role"** and often demonstrates the four elements of this role (the person is not held responsible for his or her illness, the person is expected to seek health care, the person is excused from normal social role responsibilities, the person is expected to want to get well and to cooperate). Not all sick people conform to these four sick role expectations. The **stage of convalescence** occurs when the sick person is ready to leave his or her role, usually when symptoms lessen.

People who are ill often experience various **stages of grief** as described by Kubler-Ross. **Shock or denial** is the first stage and is characterized by the inability to accept what is happening to oneself. Next, the person enters the **anger phase,** in which the person is angry that this illness is happening to oneself. The person may then move into the **bargaining stage.** In this stage the person makes promises (to God, himself, or family) in hopes of arranging a recovery. When the individual accepts the fact that he or she is ill, this is called the **depression stage.** The depression stage is characterized by sadness, crying, and fear. The final stage of the grief reaction is the **acceptance stage.** The individual learns to live with the situation during this final stage, even if this illness means a handicap or death.

It is important for nurses to be aware of Parsons's stages of illness and Kubler-Ross's stages of grief in order to understand their clients' reactions to illness as well as to help their clients to deal with illness.

Illness in an **infant** may adversely affect both the child and the parents. Babies have limited physical reserves for fighting illness, and the separation from parents may hinder the infant's ability to develop a sense of trust. Parents may lose their confidence in themselves as parents when an infant becomes ill.

The **toddler** who is ill may have difficulty in developing a sense of autonomy (independence). The ill **preschool child** may incorrectly feel that he or she is being punished for being "bad" when he or she is subjected to painful or frightening procedures.

It is often difficult for the **schoolager** who is ill to be out of school for long periods of time and to fall behind his or her peers. The **adolescent** is especially concerned about the effects of illness on his or her appearance and also needs to maintain a sense of independence.

Illness is difficult for the **young** and **middle-aged adult** to accept because these are usually one's highly productive and busy years. This individual may need repeated explanations on the importance of recommended therapies before being able to comply.

Because **older adults** are concerned about money and maintaining their independence, they are often reluctant to seek medical help. Nurses can play a major role in helping the elderly acquire health care while maintaining their independent housing needs.

Basic assumptions about illness and health include the following:

1. Illness is always a stressful situation.
2. Coming for health care is stressful.
3. Health care involves an expense.
4. Good health leads to improved health; poor health leads to worsening health.
5. It is better to keep people well than to restore wellness after they have become ill.

DRILL AND PRACTICE QUESTIONS FOR REVIEW

Complete the statements below.

1. The three stages of illness according to Parsons are _____, _____, and _____.

2. _____ and _____ are the two phases of the transition stage, according to Parsons.

3. When someone asks friends, family, and neighbors about signs and symptoms of an illness, this person is in the _____ phase of transition.

4. _____ and _____ readiness for recovery are necessary before one can return to health.

5. An individual who cannot accept that he or she has an illness, even though he or she has the symptoms, is said to be in the _____ phase of the grief reaction.

6. Mr. Jones, who has bowel cancer, has been very sad for the last few days and is now crying. He is in the _____ stage of grief.

7. An infant who is ill and separated from his or her parents may have difficulty developing a sense of _____.

8. The toddler who is ill and bedridden may have difficulty developing a sense of _____.

9. Two of the basic assumptions about illness are that illness always is a _____ situation and involves an _____.

10. _____ health leads to improved health; _____ health leads to worsening health.

Determine whether the following statements are TRUE or FALSE.

1. All people react the same way to illness.

2. The body part affected by illness may determine how soon a person seeks medical help.

3. People with poor self-esteem often perceive themselves as more susceptible to illness.

4. Lack of money and transportation are often considered barriers to seeking health care.

5. The first stage of illness is called the stage of acceptance.

6. A parent's ability to care for his or her sick child is influenced by whether or not the parent feels responsibility for the child's illness.

7. Fear is not a common reason for delaying medical advice.

8. The stages of grief usually progress in the following order: denial, anger, bargaining, depression, and acceptance.

9. It is important for nurses to meet a client's anger with anger.

10. The middle-aged adult readily accepts illness because of his or her high level of maturity.

Situation

Mr. Roberts is a forty-five-year-old insurance salesman who has had a worsening cough for two months and is now coughing blood-tinged sputum. His diagnostic tests have revealed a cancerous lung tumor. The physician has just informed Mr. Roberts of these results. Describe the stages of grief the nurse can expect Mr. Roberts to experience, and describe the ways in which the nurse can help Mr. Roberts deal with these reactions.

ANSWERS TO DRILL AND PRACTICE QUESTIONS

Completion Exercises

1. transition, acceptance, convalescence

2. Awareness, confirmation

3. confirmation

4. Physical, psychological

5. Shock (or denial)

6. depressive

7. trust

8. initiative

9. stressful, expense

10. Good, poor

True/False Exercises

1. F
2. T
3. T
4. T
5. F

6. T
7. F
8. T
9. F
10. F

Situation

Situation 1

Even though Mr. Roberts had ominous symptoms, he will likely first feel shock or denial. The nurse may have to repeat instructions and other information several times to Mr. Roberts. Because of his high stress levels during the shock stage, he has difficulty processing information.

The next stage is the anger stage. It will be difficult to care for Mr. Roberts during this stage because he will have the need to vent his anger. A useful nursing strategy would be to point out to Mr. Roberts that he seems angry and upset and then allow him ample opportunity to verbalize his anger.

Mr. Roberts may begin to bargain with God, himself, or others in an effort to arrange a better diagnosis for himself. Usually the nurse is unaware when and if a client is experiencing this bargaining stage.

Mr. Roberts may next become continually sad, may cry, may enter into the depressive stage. People who are depressed do not solve problems well; therefore, the nurse should not expect Mr. Roberts to be able to deal well with stressful situations and decisions at this time. He may begin to ask questions about his illness and the treatment plan. The nurse should answer his questions accurately but without lengthy details. Fear, which often accompanies the sad feelings, may cause Mr. Roberts to overreact to relatively minor inconveniences. The nurse should also accept his unhappy feelings and crying spells.

Finally, Mr. Roberts may accept his situation, and at this time he will be able to participate in planning care and to participate in self-care. However, he may not reach the acceptance stage until many months later.

Chapter 15

ETHNICITY AND CULTURE IN HEALTH AND ILLNESS

MAJOR NURSING CONCEPTS

Culture is a set of traditions which influence our view of the world, as well as our view of ourselves and others, and it affects one's approach to health care. **Ethnicity** is defined as the cultural group into which one is born. When one adopts cultural traditions from others, it is called **assimilation** (or acculturization). Perceiving one's own culture as better than all others is called **ethnocentrism.**

In order to give quality nursing care, nurses need to consider their clients' cultural diversity. Being able to care for clients from various cultures was termed **transcultural nursing** by a nursing leader named Leininger.

When planning their nursing care, nurses should avoid **stereotyping** (expecting people to act in a characteristic manner resulting from their cultural background) clients, to avoid inappropriate and nonindividualized care.

A thorough nursing assessment should include eight considerations pertinent to cultural differences and their health care implications. **Male and female roles** differ from culture to culture, especially with respect to whether the male or female is expected to play the dominant role. **Communication ability** refers to differences in language, accents, and dialects between the client and health care worker. Different cultures hold different values about **time orientation.** For example, Americans value punctuality, while many other cultures do not share this concern for time. Some cultures value a productive work ethic, while others place more emphasis on leisure time. This is called a **work orientation.** The **past, present, and future orientation** of your client should also be considered. Family structures vary. The **family orientation** in some cultures may include just the nuclear family, while in other cultures the extended family is the norm. **Cultural perceptions of illness** (viewing disease as caused by bacteria, evil spirits, or punishment from God) may significantly affect the way your client deals with illness and suggested treatments. **Nutritional practices** are strongly culturally related; since good nutrition is necessary for health, cultural food habits should be an essential part of the nursing assessment.

The nurse in the United States is likely to care for clients from many different cultures. Although individual differences must always be considered, it is important to study cultural aspects as a whole.

The **middle-class American** cultural orientation includes the dominant male authority figure, an attitude which has been compromised in recent years by influences of the women's movement; a strong family orientation; the Protestant work ethic; conservative views on most ideas; a value placed on higher education; materialism; a future orientation; and a belief in God. The **health problem** frequently encountered by the middle-class American are cardiovascular illness, and breast, lung, uterine, and colon cancers. Most Americans believe it is permissible for women to cry, but crying is seen as unmanly in men.

Nurses can improve their nursing care of middle-class Americans by teaching preventative health care, respecting the cost of health care, respecting American's future orientation, and carefully assessing the masked symptoms that American men frequently demonstrate in an effort to avoid socially unacceptable crying.

The **Hispanic** culture (persons of Mexican, Puerto Rican, Cuban, and other Spanish-speaking origins) is prevalent in this country. As with Americans, Hispanic individuals have certain orientations specific to their culture. The Hispanic male is expected to be "macho," a good provider for his family, and would find it difficult to accept illness and dependency. The Hispanic female is expected to be submissive and dedicated to her family. Hispanic children are expected to receive an elementary education, begin working at a young age, and follow traditional male or female roles. The families tend to be large, Spanish speaking at home, practicing the Roman Catholic faith, and oriented to the present. Persons from Hispanic cultures may delay seeking medical attention because many believe in folk medicine, herbalists (yerbero), healers (curandero), and supernatural healers (experitualistos). These alternative health providers are more attractive to the sick Hispanic because they speak Spanish and charge little or no money. Nurses can improve their nursing care to the Hispanic population by respecting and not commenting negatively about the herbalista and healers.

Spanish-speaking interpreters should be used, and adequate time should be given to the patient to confer with the large family about the treatment plan. Be aware that the average Mexican child may plot below average on the American-standardized height and weight charts. Male clients may be stoic in the face of pain, while female clients are expected to verbalize freely about their pain. Keep in mind that the male client may expect to direct how things are done.

The **Black American** is often (but not always) family oriented, values education, is religious, and is economically disadvantaged. Hypertension, tuberculosis, higher than average infant mortality rate, sickle cell anemia, and lead poisoning are major health problems prevalent in the black community. Measures to improve the delivery of health care to black Americans include providing educational experiences for young mothers, locating health care facilities near public transportation, always being respectful, and learning inner city jargon without trying to imitate it.

Native Americans are present oriented, matriarchal (female dominated), and stoic in the face of pain; the women avoid eye contact as a sign of respect. Health problems include tuberculosis, diabetes, alcoholism, high suicide rate, and inadequate immunization. The religious beliefs of Native Americans are closely interrelated with health care beliefs. Nurses can improve their nursing care of Native Americans by understanding their concern for the harmonious relationship of human and nature; offering emotional support; being careful not to mix home herbal remedies with medications since such a combination might lead to toxicity; using touch sparingly; understanding their stoicism in the face of pain; and appreciating their lack of eye contact as a sign of respect.

The **Chinese** family is patriarchal (male dominated), respectful toward elders, independent, and education-oriented. Chinese people often believe that the forces of yin and yang affect health. Acupuncture is used to treat various ailments. Health problems include tuberculosis (related to crowded living conditions), malnutrition, and dental caries (both related to poverty). Nurses can improve the health care of Chinese Americans by providing an interpreter when required, being respectful of the wishes and ideas of the older members of the family, and consulting with the dietician and family to coordinate appropriate foods.

The **Appalachian** culture is patriarchal and present oriented; education is not stressed. Appalachian people are family oriented but do not join groups because of their suspiciousness of other people. Health problems in Appalachian communities include black lung, occupational hazards (in the coal mines), and nutritionally deficient diets. Nurses can improve health care delivery for Appalachian people by gaining their acceptance before making changes, making transportation arrangements so that women and children can reach health care facilities, using touch selectively, and respecting their pride.

Southeastern Asia people have difficulty with the English language, are patriarchal, and are not time oriented. Health problems include malnutrition, dental caries, and tuberculosis. Improving health care for Asian Americans includes being respectful of differences in time orientation, omitting milk in the diet (because of digestive difficulties with milk products), and permitting unconventional visiting privileges.

In summary, it is important for nurses to respect cultural differences and to incorporate these differences into individual nursing care plans.

DRILL AND PRACTICE QUESTIONS FOR REVIEW

Complete the statements below.

1. _____ is defined as a view of the world and a set of traditions that a specific group uses and transmits to the next generation.

2. One's _____ refers to the cultural group into which one was born.

3. People in the United States who belong to ethnic groups other than the white ethnic group are usually referred to as _____.

4. When an immigrant in the United States has begun to adopt the American language, diet, and other traditions, the person is becoming _____.

5. Expecting people to act in characteristic ways without considering individual characteristics is called _____.

6. The dominant person in the Native American family is the _____.

7. The middle-class American orientation toward productive work is often termed the _____.

8. While some cultures are past oriented, Americans tend to be _____ and _____ oriented.

9. One of the major health problems affecting middle-class American men is _____.

10. People from Hispanic cultures are often nutritionally deficient in _____ and _____.

11. A type of anemia commonly seen in blacks is called _____.

12. Hypertension is a health problem seen very often in the _____ culture.

13. Native American women often avoid making eye contact as a sign of _____.

14. The _____ and _____ rate for Native Americans is higher than the average rate.

15. The dominant figure in the Chinese family is usually the _____.

Determine whether the following statements are TRUE or FALSE.

1. Ethnocentrism is a belief that your own culture is superior to all others.

2. "All Chinese children are excellent students" is a stereotypical statement.

3. Southeast Asians are extremely punctual and time oriented.

4. Middle-class Americans tend to be materialistic.

5. Spiritualists and healers should play no part in holistic nursing care.

6. The lack of roughage in the diet of many Americans is suspected to be a major factor in the cause of colon cancer.

7. Hispanic men and women are expected to verbalize freely and physically demonstrate their level of discomfort and pain.

8. Lactose deficiency is often caused by the inability of the body to digest milk because the person lacks the lactase enzyme.

9. Because of their strong family bonds, Native Americans have a lower than average infant mortality rate.

10. Nurses should incorporate the frequent use of touch in their care of an Appalachian person.

Situations

Situation 1

Mr. Bermudez is a fifty-year-old Hispanic auto mechanic who is hospitalized for a fractured pelvis. The doctor has ordered bed rest, a regular diet, and pain medications when necessary. List specific elements of your nursing care plan pertinent to Mr. Bermudez's cultural background.

Situation 2

Mrs. Lin is a seventy-two-year-old grandmother who is brought to the emergency room complaining of chest pain and shortness of breath. She is accompanied by her three children and several grandchilren. She speaks no English but occasionally converses with her eldest son in Chinese. Mrs. Lin is going to be admitted for observation. List specific elements of your nursing care plan pertinent to Mrs. Lin's cultural background.

ANSSERS TO DRILL AND PRACTICE QUESTIONS

Completion Exercises

1. Culture

2. ethnicity

3. minorities

4. assimilated (or acculturized)

5. stereotyping

6. oldest woman

7. Protestant work ethic

8. present, future

9   cardiovascular disease

10. vitamins, protein

11. sickle cell anemia

12. black American

13. respect

14. suicide, alcoholism

15. father

True/False Exercises

1.	T	6.	T
2.	T	7.	F
3.	F	8.	T
4.	T	9.	F
5.	F	10.	F

Situations

Situation 1

- Arrange for an interpreter as necessary.
- Accept any demonstrations of a "macho" attitude.
- Be aware that it will be extremely difficult for Mr. Bermudez to accept this illness and to comply with a dependent role necessitated by his bedrest.
- Arrange for a priest to visit Mr. Bermudez.
- Arrange a conference with Mr. and Mrs. Bermudez and the hospital dietician in order to provide foods which this patient will prefer.
- Begin discharge planning early because his family will readily be prepared to take over his care at home.
- Assess nonverbal cues of pain (clenched fists, rapid breathing) because Mr. Bermudez will not verbally complain of pain.
- Because of strong family ties, allow for liberal visiting hours.

Situation 2

- Allow Mrs. Lin's eldest son to stay with her and act as her interpreter.
- Understand that since her eldest son is probably the patriarch of the family, she will respect his wishes.
- Allow Mrs. Lin time to discuss with her family any treatment alternatives.
- Apprise the dietician of Mrs. Lin's cultural background so that personal food preferences will be included in her diet
- Realize that her avoidance of eye contact is a sign of respect.
- Before administering any medications to Mrs. Lin, ascertain whether she has been taking any herbal medicines at home which may interfere with or adversely affect the current medication regime.
- Be sure to demonstrate respect for Mrs. Lin as an experienced elderly person.

Chapter 16

THE IMPACT OF STRESS ON HEALTH

MAJOR NURSING CONCEPTS

When exposed to **stressors** (physiological or psychological threats), the body reacts to protect itself and maintain a state of physiological balance (**homeostasis**) through physiological stress responses or the General Adaptation Syndrome. These responses are part of **coping** (immediate response of a person to a stressor) and **adaptation** (ultimate change that occurs in a person as a result of the stressor). Adaptation is physiologic and psychologic, takes time, varies from person to person, depends on negative feedback, may be inadequate or exaggerated, and/or can be exhausting and fail.

The **General Adaptation Syndrome** includes the **alarm stage** (body prepares to defend itself); the **stage of resistance** (adaptive body changes occur in response to the stressor to maintain homeostasis); and, if the body's ability to resist the stressor wears out, the **stage of exhaustion** (death). Stress responses are involuntary and mediated by the sympathetic nervous system. Essentially, these responses are aimed at mobilizing the body to defend itself against the stressor (fight or flight responses). The continued presence of a stressor initiates parasympathetic activity that can precipitate health problems, such as peptic ulcer disease. The more damaging a stressor is (or the extent to which the stressor is perceived as damaging by the person), the more difficult adaptation will be. When stressors persist or more than one stressor is experienced, the more difficult adaptation will be. The presence of support persons or experience in dealing with a particular stressor facilitates adaptation.

Psychological adaptation also occurs in response to stressors. It is manifested as **anxiety** (behavior that occurs in response to an unknown theat). Anxiety can be kept at a minimum by using **coping mechanisms**. These include **approach** (actively dealing with the stressor), **withdrawal** (avoidance of the stressor), or **inaction** (consciously deciding not to react to the stressor). People with Type A personalities place themselves under constant stress and are more predisposed, therefore, to stress-related health problems.

When an individual's psychological coping abilities are no longer effective in alleviating a feeling of stress (e.g., when stress is long-term), the individual is in a state of **crisis**. Crises may be **maturational** (accompanies developmental changes) or **situational** (accompanies an unexpected event). In dealing with a crisis, a person utilizes a known, effective coping mechanism to help alleviate her or his anxiety. If this process fails, a back-up solution is tried. Nurses serve as support persons for individuals, especially when crises remain unresolved. The ability of individuals to problem-solve and cope with crises varies with age.

Assessments that reflect an individual dealing with stress are varied and include cognitive (planned), verbal, and motor (action) responses. **Cognitive responses** include increasing one's knowledge about the stressor, problem-solving, structuring (arranging a situation so that stressors are less likely to occur), exerting self-control, dreaming and fantasizing, suppression, and prayer. **Verbal responses** include talking, crying, laughing, screaming, and verbal abuse. **Motor responses** include hitting and kicking, touching, running, and hyperventilation. Individuals may use mental **defense mechanisms** such as **denial, rationalization** (substituting a nonthreatening solution for a threatening one); **intellectualization** (talking about a situation as if not personally involved); **identification** (assuming the characteristics of another person); **reaction formation** (acting the opposite of one's true feelings); **repression** (excluding an idea from conscious thought); **projection** (transferring feelings to another person); **compensation** (carrying out an activity other than the one desired); **regression** (adopting behavior from an earlier life stage); and **sublimation** (transforming unacceptable drives to more acceptable behaviors). People who are losing their coping abilities in dealing with a stressor may demonstrate disorganized, repetitive, or unusual behavior. They may be less aware of environmental happenings, misinterpret reality, experience poor memory, have a lessened self-esteem, and experience psychosomatic symptoms.

A **nursing diagnosis** that specifically pertains to stress is:

- Coping
- Ineffective.

Planning and implementation strategies to alleviate stress include helping people learn successful coping strategies, offering support, and **crisis intervention.** Crisis intervention is a problem-solving technique that includes identification of the problem, listing of alternative solutions, choosing from among alternative solutions, implementation of the chosen solution, and evaluation of the success of the solution.

Unresolved crisis situations can result in **burnout** (physical and emotional exhaustion, negative self-concept and attitude, loss of concern for others), drug and/or alcohol dependence, accidents, violence, abuse, and suicide.

DRILL AND PRACTICE QUESTIONS FOR REVIEW

Complete the statements below.

1. The term that represents a less static state of body balance than homeostasis is _____.

2. During the alarm stage of the GAS, the _____ nervous system initiates responses.

3. The stages of the GAS include: _____, _____, and _____.

4. An individual who has hemorrhaged has managed to maintain an adequate BP. Suddenly, his BP falls, despite the fact that bleeding has stopped. He is probably in the _____ stage of the GAS.

5. The psychological state that occurs in response to an unknown threat is _____; the state that occurs in response to a known threat is _____.

6. A person experiences the death of a loved one. This can precipitate a _____ crisis.

7. Coping mechanisms for dealing with stress include _____, _____, and _____.

8. Problem-solving ability emerges in the child during the end of the _____ year.

9. The increased respiratory rate associated with acute stress is called _____.

10. The problem-solving process used in helping people resolve crises is called _____.

11. Drug dependence can involve _____ and/or _____ dependence.

12. Alcohol and opiates are central nervous system _____.

Determine whether the following statements are TRUE or FALSE.

1. In general, during the alarm stage of the GAS, body processes are speeded up.

2. In response to an oncoming car, an individual is energized to run quickly as a result of involuntary stress responses.

3. Adaptation to a stressor involves physiological and psychological responses.

4. Adaptation responses are predictable from person to person.

5. Adaptive responses are always beneficial.

6. The longer a person must continue to deal with a stressor, the more effective stress responses become.

7. Similar events evoke similar stress responses among all individuals.

8. As a person becomes more anxious, he or she is more likely to concentrate on details.

9. The birth of a child is not considered a stressful event because it is a pleasant, happy occasion.

10. When confronted with a situational crisis, crying should be discouraged.

11. Screaming should be discouraged as a means of releasing tension.

12. A deterioration in ability to organize may indicate that a person is experiencing stress.

13. Memory becomes more acute as stress increases.

Match each of the defense mechanisms in Column A with a representative example from Column B.

Column A	Column B
1. regression	a. a parent who is angry with a child goes jogging to release tension
2. intellectualization	b. a child resumes drinking from a bottle when as sibling is born
3. identification	c. a mother discusses the accident that killed her child as if she were discussing the death of an unknown person
4. reaction formation	d. a person braggs a lot about her accomplishments but really has a poor self-concept
5. sublimation	e. a child imitates his father

Situations

Situation 1

Juan Lopez has just suffered a severe injury. Provide assessments of Juan that would suggest he was in the alarm stage of the GAS.

Situation 2

Mary Jones, RN, is aware of the potential for experiencing burnout. Discuss ways she can prevent burnout from occurring.

Situation 3

As a school nurse, you frequently talk with adolescents. Provide assessments suggesting that a particular adolescent might be contemplating suicide.

ANSWERS TO DRILL AND PRACTICE QUESTIONS

Completion Exercises

1. homeodynamics
2. sympathetic
3. alarm, resistance, exhaustion
4. exhaustion
5. anxiety, fear
6. situational
7. approach, withdrawal, inaction
8. first
9. hyperventilation
10. crisis intervention
11. physical, psychic
12. depressants

True/False Exercises

1.	T	7.	F
2.	T	8.	T
3.	T	9.	F
4.	F	10.	F
5.	F	11.	F
6.	F	12.	T
		13.	F

Matching

1. b
2. c
3. e
4. d
5. a

Situations

Situation 1

Assessments indicating that Juan is in alarm stage of GAS:

- increase in heart rate, respiratory rate, and BP
- diaphoresis
- dilated pupils
- pallor
- decreased urine output

Situation 2

To prevent burnout, she can

- avoid contact with burned-out persons or ask them to avoid expressing their negative attitudes while they are with her
- avoid boredom and routine by doing different things or doing the same things differently
- stay healthy by having adequate diet and sleep
- reward herself

Situation 3

Assessments that suggest adolescent's potential for suicide:

- talks about suicide
- describes a suicide plan
- lacks a successful psychological support system
- has history of suicide attempt
- has had recent exposure to suicide attempt or actual suicide of a friend or family member
- shows alcohol/drug abuse
- has had change in attitude from sad to happy

PART V

THE NURSE AS CAREGIVER AND HEALTH PROMOTER

Chapter 17

MEETING HEALTH CARE NEEDS ACROSS THE LIFE SPAN:
CONCEPTION THROUGH SCHOOL AGE

MAJOR NURSING CONCEPTS

Growth refers to an increase in a person's physical size, while **development** is defined as an increase in a person's cognitive and behavioral functions. Growth and development are active, continuous, and orderly processes which vary in rate from person to person. **Genetic** and **environmental** factors, such as **sex, health, intelligence, nutritional status,** and **socioeconomic** status , influence growth and development. Physical and mental **handicaps** interfere with normal growth and development to varying degrees.

The nurse is concerned with the growth and development of persons **throughout the lifespan,** from conception to/and including dying and death. When assessing growth and development, the nurse needs to consider the following: life stages, measurements of physical growth, measurements of developmental functions, measurements of intelligence levels, risk factors prevalent in each age group, and psychosocial aspects.

Sigmund Freud identified stages of development for different age groups and used these stages to relate childhood experiences to later mental problems.

Erik Erikson described developmental steps in humans encompassing eight identified life stages (see Table 17-2). Accomplishment of level tasks at each stage leads to individual fulfillment. Because health promotion measures vary according to age, nurses need to be familiar with these level tasks and the health maintenance procedures recommended for each age group.

Stages of cognitive and intellectual development were defined by **Jean Piaget.**

Intrauterine (embryo and fetal) growth and development and health promotion include the provision for adequate nutrition (delivered to the fetus via the **placenta**) and protection from **teratogens** (substances detrimental to embryo growth). The movement of the fetus felt by the mother is referred to as **quickening.**

The **neonate's** (first four weeks of life) cardiorespiratory status, muscle tone, reflex activity, and color are rated using an **Apgar** score. Additional nursing assessments of **vernix caseosa** (thick white skin covering), **lanugo** (fine downy hair across shoulders), **milla** (white lesions across nose), **physiological jaundice** (yellow color to skin), and **meconium** (black first stool) are specific to the neonate.

Efforts to foster **parent-child bonding** are an important part of your nursing care plan. **Birthing rooms** (a relaxed "at-home" atmosphere in the hospital setting) and **rooming-in** (hospital policy that allows infants to be cared for by their parents) permit parents to spend time with their newborn and facilitates parent-child bonding. Separation of a newborn from the parents because of illness interferes with parent-child bonding. Nursing interventions such as unrestricted visiting hours and involving the parents in the ill newborn's care are encouraged.

Assessment of the **infant** (1 to 12 months) should emphasize physical examination and the use of developmental tests such as the **Denver Developmental Screening Test.** Physical growth is rapid, and developmental events are multiple. Freud refers to the infant period as the **oral stage.** During the first year, the child develops a **sense of trust.** Erikson describes trust as learning to love and be loved. An infant develops a sense of trust when his or her needs are consistently and lovingly met. **Nursing interventions** are aimed at providing adequate **nutrition** (primarily milk, cereals, and strained foods) and **rest** (sixteen hours out of twenty-four), **promoting skin integrity** (preventing diaper rash), and the **prevention of accidents.**

Common health problems occurring during the infancy period are **night bottle syndrome** (extensive tooth decay from prolonged contact with sweetened milk), **diaper rash, seborrheic dermatitis** (cradle cap), **colic** (sharp intermittent abdominal pain), and **teething pain.**

Physical and mental **handicaps** (conditions that interfere with normal psychologic or physical functioning) may hinder parent-child bonding, developmental progress, and the acquisition of the sense of trust.

The **toddler** (one to three years) begins to demonstrate **independence** (self-feeding, self-dressing, self-toileting). Erikson refers to this period of independence as the time when the child develops a **sense of autonomy versus shame and doubt.** Freud calls the toddler stage the **anal stage.** Piaget describes the toddler as experiencing the **sensorimotor stage** of cognitive development.

It is more difficult for the **handicapped toddler** to achieve a sense of autonomy because physical and mental limitations may foster dependence rather than independence.

The rate of physical growth, appetite, and number of sleeping hours decrease during this stage. special considerations for the care of the **toddler** include **toilet training**(at age three most children have achieved adequate cephalocaudal and cognitive development to master toilet training), **prevention of accidents** (falls, poisoning), handling **temper tantrums** and **negativism** (answering *no* to every question).

Ritualism (some actions done the same way every day) fosters reassurance and a sense of security.

The **preschooler** (three to six years) learns new skills very rapidly but is in a slow physical growth period. Freud describes this stage as the **phallic stage** in which the **Electra complex**(a girl begins to compete with the mother for love of the father) and the **Oedipus complex** (a boy competes with the father for the mother's love) originate. Achieving a **sense of initiative versus guilt** is the goal of the preschool period, as defined by Erikson. Piaget sees preschool children in the **preoperational period** (being able to master only very simple problem-solving) of cognitive development

The **handicapped preschooler** has a special need to develop problem-solving skills in order to acquire a sense of initiative. Simple activities (walking, feeding, talking, may be difficult.

Health maintenance concerns for the preschooler include **sleep disturbance** due to fears and nightmares, **nutritional deficits** because of a decreased appetite, **safety,** exposure to **upper respiratory infections,** and **nonfluency** (language pattern similar to stuttering). **Tall-tale telling** refers to the untrue stories that preschoolers relate. The child is not intentionally lying but rather is replying to a question with an answer he or she thinks will be most pleasing. It is important to keep this phenomenon in mind when asking preschoolers important questions about pain, medicine, or substances they may have eaten.

For the **school-ager** (six to twelve years), growth at the beginning of this stage is slow, but near the end of this stage growth and development begin to spurt. **Secondary sexual characteristics** such as pubic and auxiliary hair and breast changes appear, marking the onset of puberty. **Menarche** refers to the beginning of menstruation in girls.

Freud did not consider this period important to mental health and referred to it as the **latent period.** Erikson describes the developmental goals of this period as achieving a **sense of industry versus inferiority.** During the school-age years, children learn to do things well. They function at the **operational level** of cognition, according to Piaget.

Learning to do things well promotes a sense of industry. Therefore it is important for *handicapped school-agers* to participate in activities that they can complete satisfactorily.

Health promotion activities for the school-ager focus on **accident prevention** (avoiding sports injuries and street accidents), **dental care, personal hygiene,** adequate **nutrition** (protein, calcium, vitamin D, low fat), **rest** (eight to ten hours), and **exercise,** and the **avoidance of substance abuse.** Additional concerns for the school-ager include physical problems such as **scoliosis** (sideways curvature of the spine) and **sinus headaches** as well as social problems such as **school phobia** and **stealing.** School-agers who lack adult supervision for part of each day are referred to as **latchkey children.**

When using the nursing process to meet health care needs from conception through school-age, some commonalities are evident. **Nursing assessments** include measurements of growth and development. **Nursing diagnoses** for the pregnancy period include individual and family coping; and for the newborn and infant include diagnoses related to health maintenance. In the toddler, preschooler, and school-ager, the potential for injury is an important nursing diagnosis. **Nursing interventions** focus on promoting developmental tasks, fostering physical growth, and the prevention of illness and accidents.

DRILL AND PRACTICE QUESTIONS FOR REVIEW

Complete the statements below.

1. In order to measure growth, recording an infant's _____ and _____ is an essential part of a basic nursing assessment.

2. The placenta supplies _____ and _____ to the growing fetus.

3. The _____, _____, and _____ are tissue layers in the developing embryo.

4. Substances hazardous to embryotic growth are called _____.

5. Immediately after birth, newborns are assessed for general cardiorespiratory function by an _____ score.

6. _____ is the thick black first stool of the newborn.

7. The leading cause of death in infants and toddlers is _____.

8. Because the toddler is concerned with toilet training, Freud called this stage the _____ stage.

9. According to Erikson, handicapped and nonhandicapped children develop a sense of _____ during the toddler period.

10. Preschool children often develop a language pattern similar to stuttering known as _____.

11. The initial onset of menstruation is called _____.

12. The school-ager's diet needs to contain adequate amounts of _____, _____, and _____ for tissue and bone growth.

13. Cognitive and intellectual development were studied and defined by _____.

14. _____ is the term used to describe fetal movement felt by the mother.

15. Children who have periods of unsupervised time are called _____.

Determine whether the following statements are TRUE or FALSE.

1. A newborn's behavior should be rated, using the Brazelton Behavioral Scale, within the first forty-eight hours after delivery.

2. The Denver Developmental Screening Test determines a toddler's intelligence level.

3. The vernix caseosa is a protective cheesy white substance covering a newborn's skin.

4. Newborns normally sleep ten to twelve out of every twenty-four hours.

5. Cuddling and comforting an infant after a painful nursing procedure is nice but not important.

6. Thumb-sucking during the first year of life should be discouraged.

7. A toddler who has accidently swallowed lye should be given Ipecac.

8. Toddlers normally have hearty appetites.

9. A two-year-old may have twenty deciduous teeth.

10. Most children are physiologically and cognitively ready for toilet training at three years of age.

11. Health screening for school-agers includes tests for scoliosis and serum cholesterol levels.

12. Substance abuse is practically nonexistent in grade-school children.

13. Freud did not consider the school-age years important to mental health.

14. According to Piaget, school-age children function at the operational level of cognition.

15. It is a good idea for handicapped school-agers to participate in difficult activities even if they cannot accomplish the tasks.

Situations

Situation 1

Mrs. Smith is a twenty-eight-year-old woman who has just been told by her physician that she is two months pregnant. This is Mrs. Smith's first pregnancy. While interacting with this client, what specific factors would the nurse include in the teaching plan in an effort to enhance fetal growth and development?

Situation 2

As a school nurse, you are planning a health teaching program for children ages ten to twelve years (the school-ager). List the appropriate topics you would include in your plan.

ANSWERS TO DRILL AND PRACTICE QUESTIONS

Completion Exercises

1. height, weight
2. oxygen, nutrients
3. mesoderm, entoderm, ectoderm
4. teratogens
5. Apgar
6. meconium
7. accidents
8. anal
9. autonomy or independence
10. nonfluency
11. menarche
12. protein, calcium, vitamin D
13. Jean Piaget
14. Quickening
15. latchkey children

True/False Exercises

1. F
2. F
3. T
4. F
5. F
6. F
7. F
8. F
9. T
10. T
11. T
12. F
13. T
14. T
15. F

Situations

Situation 1

- include the husband in teaching sessions
- provide for adequate nutrition for the mother and child
- emphasize the importance of prenatal check-ups
- indicate no smoking
- indicate avoidance of alcohol
- emphasize that no medication be taken without primary health care provider's approval
- consider the adjustment to psychosocial aspects of pregnancy

Situation 2

The health teaching program should include

- accident prevention
- dental care
- development of secondary sexual characteristics• exercise and rest
- nutrition
- personal hygiene
- substance abuse

Chapter 18

MEETING HEALTH CARE NEEDS ACROSS THE LIFESPAN:
THE ADOLESCENT AND ADULT YEARS

MAJOR NURSING CONCEPTS

A person grows to physical and psychological maturity during **adolescence** (twelve to eighteen years).

Rapid physical growth during adolescence is evidence by **increases** in **height** and **weight.** As during other growth spurts, the adolescent requires adequate **sleep** (approximately ten hours each night), **nutrition** (diet high in protein, calcium, and vitamin D, and iron supplements for menstruating girls). A daily **exercise** program is an important part of an adolescent's health plan.

Changes in **secondary sexual characteristics** continue until maturity is reached. An objective instrument used to measure sexual maturity is the **Tanner Stages of Maturity Scale.** Changes in the vital signs, such as an increasing blood pressure and decreasing pulse and respiratory rates, proceed until adult levels are reached.

Developmentally, Sigmund **Freud** described adolescence as the **genital period** and believed an adolescent's activities are ruled by the **libido** (sexual influences).

According to Erik **Erikson,** the goal of adolescence is to gain a sense of **identity versus role confusion.** In order to eliminate role confusion and achieve a sense of identity, the adolescent progresses through several sequential steps. **Establishing a value system** is the first step, which refers to a sense of what one believes in or values. **Adjusting to a new body image** is the next step, which includes the process of getting acquainted with the many physical changes that adolescents experience. Making decisions on one's own is an important step, which is called **emancipation from parents.** Learning to deal with others from a male or female perspective and not as a child is the step Erikson describes as **establishing heterosexual relationships.** Finally, **making a vocational choice** refers to the often difficult decision-making process about one's life vocation.

Cognitive development during the adolescent period reaches the adult level. However, adolescents often experience problem-solving difficulties because of their exposure to varied and frequent stressors. Adolescents do not always reason well.

Handicapped adolescents experience difficulty in several developmental areas such as their sense of identity, choosing a vocation, emancipation from parents, making decisions for themselves, and establishing heterosexual relationships.

Safety is a major concern for all adolescents. **Motor vehicle** (including motorcycle) **accidents** are the major cause of death in adolescents. **Anorexia nervosa** (refusal to eat) and **bulimia** (food binges accompanied by forced vomiting), **peptic ulcers, obesity, sexually transmitted diseases** (gonorrhea, syphilis, herpes simplex II, AIDS), **adolescent pregnancy, acne** (acne vulgaris), and **suicide** are additional health problems frequently seen in the adolescent population.

Health care measures should include the teaching of **routine testicular examination** for boys and **breast examination** for girls. Because adolescents are present-oriented, effective health teaching is best directed at immediate concerns. For example, discussing immediate rewards such as shiny hair, clear skin, and a small waistline as an outcome of sound nutrition is preferable to discussing far distant outcomes.

Young adulthood (eighteen to forty-five years) is a busy and often stressful period. Career decisions are made final, home management begins, higher education is sought, and childbearing and child-rearing occur during these years. Physical endurance is at its peak, and it is the ideal time for childbearing. Sexual maturity is reached. Some people continue to grow an additional inch or two in early young adulthood.

Developmentally, **Erikson** refers to these years as the **intimacy versus isolation period.** Intimacy, according to Erikson, is the ability to relate deeply with others through various relationships (marriage, friendships). Before one can offer deep friendship or love, he or she needs a strong sense of identity. Cognitively, young adults have mature reasoning and thought processes, and during this period they develop experience in problem-solving.

Young adults with **handicaps** find it more difficult to establish the lasting relationship necessary for achieving a sense of intimacy. They need strong support systems in order to feel good enough about themselves to reach out to others for friendship and love.

Physical requirements during this period include eight hours of **sleep** a night, a low fat **diet** adequate in protein and vitamin C, and **daily exercise.** This period is usually a healthy time of life with the exception of accidents. The high incidence of **motor vehicle accidents** persists into early adulthood.

Decisions about higher education needs and career are difficult because of the many choices available to men and women today. A sense of independence for the young adult is usually determined by the person's financial independence and ability to live away from home. Successful marriage, childbearing, and parenthood during this period require sound decision-making abilities, personal adjustment, and a strong sense of responsibility.

During the **middle-aged adult years** (forty-five to sixty-four years) primary involvement with families changes to more **community involvement.** Physically, middle-aged adults experience decreases in activity and stamina, and also tend to gain weight because of a decrease in the metabolism rate.

Both males and females undergo changes related to decreases in sex hormones. **Menopause** is the cessation of ovulation and the end of menstrual cycles in women. **Vasomotor changes** ("hot flashes"), heart palpitations, headaches, dizziness, increased risk for **osteoporosis** (loss of calcium from bone), and decreased vaginal secretions are physical changes associated with decreased estrogen levels during and after menopause. The middle-aged adult male experiences the **climacteric** or **andropause** (lessening sexual activity). Andropause symptoms are less overt. The achievement of an erection and ejaculation may take longer after men have reached the age of fifty or sixty.

Many middle-aged adults need reading glasses to correct **presbyopia** (decreased power of accommodation). The ability to hear high-pitched sounds decreases. **Arteriosclerosis** (hardening of the arteries), hypertension, and coronary artery disease develop in many people during the middle-adult years.

A **sense of generativity** (concern that goes beyond self and family and into the community) is established during the middle-aged adult years (**Erikson**). People with a sense of generativity participate in community and political activities, while people without a sense of generativity stagnate or become self-absorbed.

Participating in community and political activities which require little physical movement (answering phones, stuffing envelopes) offer excellent opportunities for the **handicapped** to develop self-esteem while at the same time broadening their social contacts.

The middle-aged adult requires approximately six to eight hours of **sleep** each night. The health care plan should include a **diet** of reduced calories and low in fats, **regular exercise, no smoking,** and **conservative alcohol consumption.**

Health care measures should include once-a-month self-breast examinations and a *Pap test* (Papanicolaou smear) every three years for women, and once-a-month testicular self-examinations for men.

During this period many people experience bouts of **depression** as shown by loss of appetite, fatigue, loss of self-esteem, neglect of personal hygiene, and expressions of sadness. The degree of depression needs to be determined so that appropriate help can be provided.

Middle-aged adults often find themselves in a situation called the **"generation gap"** (difficulty that children and parents experience in relating to each other because of a generational age difference) or in a changing marriage. Some marriages end at this time, while others start anew. Middle-aged adults also encounter the responsibilities and stress of caring for and making arrangements for ill parents.

DRILL AND PRACTICE QUESTIONS FOR REVIEW

Complete the statements below.

1. The _____ is a scale used for measuring sexual maturity.

2. Pulse and respiratory rates _____ during adolescence.

3. Freud refers to the adolescence period as the _____ period.

4. Erikson's developmental task for the adolescent is achieving a sense of _____ versus _____.

5. Menstruating females have a need for _____ supplements.

6. The major cause of death during adolescence is _____.

7. _____ is often associated with obesity in the adolescent.

8. A disease characterized by a refusal to eat is called _____.

9. _____ refers to episodes of eating binges accompanied by forced vomiting.

10. The four most common sexually transmitted diseases are _____, _____, _____, and _____.

11. The most frequently abused drug is _____.

12. The physically ideal period for childbearing is the _____.

13. The metabolism rate decreases during the _____.

14. _____ is the end of ovulation.

15. A common vision disorder requiring reading glasses in the middle-aged is called
    _____.

16. _____ is the term used to describe fatty deposits on the inner lining of the blood
    vessels.

17. According to Erikson, the older middle-aged adult begins to focus his or her attention
    away from _____ and _____ and becomes involved in
    _____ activities.

Determine whether the following statements are TRUE or FALSE.

1. Adolescent pregnancy is not traumatic for the adolescent father.

2. The second leading cause of death in the late adolescent is suicide.

3. Adolescence is a time of easy adjustment.

4. According to Freud, sexual influences are termed genital forces.

5. According to Erikson, the first step adolescents work through in order to achieve a sense
   of identity is establishing a value system.

6. Because adolescents are capable of formal operational thought, they reason very well.

7. Adolescents are future-oriented.

8. Techniques for self-breast examinations and testicular examinations should be taught to
   adolescents.

9. Long-term stress in the adolescent may precipitate peptic ulcers.

10. Effective treatment for AIDS is unknown.

11. The birth rate among adolescent girls is declining.

12. Effective treatment for acne vulgaris includes vitamin A and antibiotics.

13. A woman's sexual interest peaks during late adolescence.

14. The average young adult needs approximately ten hours of sleep each night.

15. Adolescents should begin diets low in cholesterol.

16. Ejaculation in middle-aged men is referred to as the climacteric.

17. Men are able to father children after andropause.

18. The Pap test is used to determine the presence of uterine cancer.

Situation

Mrs. Gonzales is a fifty-year-old woman who has recently relocated to your city. She
registers at the HMO (health maintenance organization) where you work. During this initial
visit, Mrs. Gonzales tells you that she has always been healthy and has not seen a doctor
for years. Describe specific factors that should be included in your health teaching plan for
Mrs. Gonzales.

ANSWERS TO DRILL AND PRACTICE QUESTIONS

Completion Exercises

1. Tanner Stages of Maturity Scale
2. slow or decrease
3. genital
4. identity, role confusion
5. iron
6. accidents
7. hypertension
8. anorexia nervosa
9. Bulimia
10. gonorrhea, syphillis, herpes simplex II, and AIDS
11. alcohol
12. young adulthood period
13. middle-aged adult period
14. Menopause
15. presbyopia
16. Arteriosclerosis
17. self, family, community

True/False Exercises

1.	T	10.	T
2.	T	11.	F
3.	F	12.	T
4.	F	13.	F
5.	T	14.	F
6.	F	15.	T
7.	F	16.	F
8.	T	17.	T
9.	T	18.	T

Situation

1. low fat, reduced calorie diet
2. no smoking
3. moderate alcohol consumption
4. regular exercise
5. Pap test every three years
6. monthly self-breast examination
7. regular eye examination
8. annual blood pressure examination for hypertension

Chapter 19

MEETING HEALTH CAE NEEDS ACROSS THE LIFE SPAN: THE LATE ADULT YEARS

MAJOR NURSING CONCEPTS

The science of aging is called **gerontology; geriatrics** refers to the health care and treatment of older persons. Nurses are expected to give holistic gerontological care to many individuals, since the **average man's life expectancy** today is **72 years** and the **average woman's life expectancy** is **77 years.**

The **aging process** is poorly understood, but it is thought to be affected by **individual biological time clocks, endocrine changes, decreased blood supply** to tissues and organs, and **changes in RNA and DNA synthesis.** Because each person ages differently, nursing assessments of the aged are done on an **individual basis.**

Decreases in **gastrointestinal function** during the late adult years include digestion difficulties, constipation, nausea and vomiting, and heartburn. Eating slowly and including fiber in the diet may eliminate these problems. Older adults may prevent dry mouth and **halitosis** (bad breath) with frequent oral hygiene and sucking on candy or ice chips.

A **decreased vital capacity** and reduced blood flow through the lungs causes fatigue and increased incidence of respiratory infections in older adults. Nursing interventions to prevent respiratory infections include deep breathing and coughing after surgery and determining the appropriateness of influenza and pneumonia vaccines.

Atherosclerosis (fatty deposits on the inner lining of blood vessels), which may become marked during the late adult years, leads to increases in pulse and blood pressure, and inadequate oxygen supply to the organs. Older adults frequently experience **orthostatic hypotension** (a sudden decrease in blood pressure due to position change) that may cause dizziness and fainting. Because of vascular changes in the legs, older adults may develop **varicose veins** (weakened veins), **intermittent claudication** (pain with walking), edema, and weak peripheral pulses. Nurses can teach clients circulation-promoting techniques such as using support hose, frequent position changes, and the avoidance of tight clothing.

Neurological changes in the older adult include slower physical and mental reaction times, hearing loss, visual problems such as **hyperopia** (poor near vision), and diminished pain sensation.

Kidney function during the late adult years decreases and may result in fluid and electrolyte imbalances and drug intoxication. Bladder tone and capacity also decrease and may lead to urgency, frequency, nocturia, and **stress incontinence** (involuntary voiding of urine when laughing, coughing, sneezing). Men who experience difficulty starting or maintaining a urine stream may have a benign or a cancerous enlargement of the prostate (**prostatic hypertrophy).**

Integument (skin and nails) changes, such as the development of dry, delicate skin, require special considerations. Nursing care should emphasize the prevention of skin breakdown. Shoes that fit well and padding of boney prominences promote skin integrity. Moisturizers, air humidifiers, and limited use of soap help prevent excessive dryness. Bleeding or nonhealing skin lesions may indicate **skin cancer.**

Older adults need daily activities; and they require calcium, vitamin D, and flouride in their diets to diminish **osteoporosis** (porous, brittle, and easily broken bones). The swelling and pain in arthritic joints is more pronounced in the morning and on rainy or cold days.

Older adult women are capable of achieving orgasm, and older males, erection and ejaculation. Although the older woman is no longer fertile after menopause, the older male remains fertile through his life.

According to Erik **Erikson,** the older adult's task is to achieve a **sense of integrity** (feeling fulfilled and worthwhile) **versus a sense of despair** (feeling that one's life has been a failure. **Life review** is the practice of an older adult telling the same story repeatedly, usually because this experience was especially rewarding.

Disengagement theory by **Cummings and Henry** refers to society's withdrawal from older adults while the older adult also withdraws from society. Supporters of this theory believe social programs for the aging are unnecessary. **Havighurst and Maddox** however, believing that activity is healthful for older adults, support programs for the aging. Others believe each person should be considered on an individual basis.

The **handicapped** older adult may feel satisfied with his or her life (sense of integrity) or may not. The absence of support people often defeats this sense of integrity.

When developing health care plans for the older adult, it is important to **incorporate the client's ideas,** wishes, and established habits. Interactions should be **respectful** and should take into consideration **memory loss.** Providing **social conversation** and some appropriate use of **touch** (such as hand-holding) are usually enjoyable to the older adult.

Older adults are encouraged to participate in **sports activities, consume fewer calories,** and avoid napping if this interferes with **sleeping** at night (approximately six hours of sleep are needed each night).

Older adults often have **financial worries** which deter them from seeking medical help, prevent adequate nutrition, housing and clothing and discourage social interactions. These factors result in poor physical health and decreased self-esteem.

Many older adult women and men experience the **death of a spouse. Grief** is a process which begins with the **initial adjustment** to the loss (about six weeks) and culminates at about two years with **final resolution.** Widows and widowers are advised not to make any major life changes for at least six months after the death of a spouse.

Safety concerns for the older adult include poor vision, hearing impairments, falls, and burns (from hot water or heating pads). Psychosocial concerns may involve adjustment to retirement, loss of a loved one, or caring for an ill spouse. Poor hygiene, disorientation, withdrawal from people and activities, and memory loss are characteristics of **depression.**

DRILL AND PRACTICE QUESTIONS FOR REVIEW

Complete the statements below.

1. The science of aging is called _____, while _____ refers to the health care and treatment of older persons.

2. The average man's life expectancy is _____ years, and the average woman's life expectancy is _____.

3. _____ is bad breath.

4. In order to avoid constipation, the older adult should eat a diet rich in _____ and _____.

5. _____ is an example of a natural laxative.

6. Older adults often develop _____, which is the accumulation of fatty deposits along the inner lining of blood vessels.

7. Leg pain with walking is called _____.

8. Older adults may experience drug intoxication and/or fluid and electrolyte imbalances because of decreased _____ function.

9. Involuntary voiding due to laughing, coughing, or sneezing is referred to as _____.

10. _____ is overgrowth of the prostate gland.

11. Three techniques nurses can use to prevent excessive skin dryness in older adults are _____, _____, and _____.

12. Skin lesions which bleed and/or do not heal may be a sign of _____.

13. _____ is a condition characterized by porous, brittle, and easily broken bones.

14. The habit of retelling about a rewarding experience over and over again is named _____.

15. The developmental task of the older adult is to achieve _____.

Determine whether the following statements are TRUE or FALSE.

1. Today one out of every fifteen people is over age sixty-five.

2. The physical and psychosocial aging processes are clearly understood today.

3. Gastrointestinal changes that occur with aging include increased peristalsis and increased enzyme action.

4. In older adults, activity may cause elevations in blood pressure.

5. Orthostatic hypotension may occur when an older adult moves from a sitting to a standing position.

6. Varicosities refer to the thickening of arterial walls in the lower legs.

7. Males who have difficulty initiating the urinary stream should seek medical attention.

8. Long term sun exposure increases one's risk for the development of skin cancer.

9. Immobility aids in the development of osteoporosis.

10. Older adult men and older adult women are infertile.

11. Older adult men and older adult women continue to enjoy sex and achieve orgasm.

12. Handicapped older adults often have difficulty achieving a sense of integrity because of the loss of support people over the years.

13. Because of their decreased sensation to pain, older adults need to increase bath water temperature and heating pad temperature.

14. Calling an older adult by nicknames such as "Pops" or "Honey" is endearing and should be encouraged.

15. Because of Medicare, Social Security, and pensions, older adults today have few financial problems.

Situation

Mrs. Walker is a seventy-seven-year-old widow hospitalized for a fractured hip. It is five days after Mrs. Walker's surgery, and she is having a good postoperative course. You are the nurse assigned to care for Mrs. Walker today. List several components of nursing care specific to the older adult which you will want to consider when caring for Mrs. Walker.

ANSWERS TO DRILL AND PRACTICE QUESTIONS

Completion Exercises

1. gerontology, geriatrics
2. seventy-two, seventy-seven
3. halitosis
4. roughage, fluids
5. prune juice
6. atherosclerosis
7. intermittent claudication
8. kidney
9. stress incontinence
10. prostatic hypertrophy
11. moisturizers, air humidifiers, limited use of soap
12. skin cancer
13. Osteoporosis
14. life review
15. a sense of integrity

True/False Exercises

1.	T	8.	T
2.	F	9	T
3.	F	10.	F
4.	T	11.	T
5.	T	12.	T
6.	F	13.	F
7.	T	14.	F
		15.	F

Situation

- Demonstrate respect for Mrs. Walker in your conversation and actions.
- Frequent reminders may be necessary.
- Incorporate the client's ideas into your nursing care plan.
- Be aware that Mrs. Walker may have financial problems.
- Use touch appropriately, such as hand-holding.
- Allow sufficient time for all activities, since older adults fatigue easily.
- Try to schedule time with Mrs. Walker for social conversation.
- Limit amount of soap in bath.
- Encourage Mrs. Walker to cough and deep breathe.
- Orient client frequently to time, day, and place.
- Be aware of safety considerations such as orthostatic hypotension, poor vision, diminished pain sensation.

Chapter 20

GRIEVING AND THE MEANING OF LOSS

MAJOR NURSING CONCEPTS

Grieving (mourning) is a psychological state that accompanies a loss (death, robbery, divorce, or unemployment). According to **Kubler-Ross** (1969) the five stages of grief are as follows:

- **Denial:** People may feel numb or shocked, and are unwilling to talk about the loss.
- **Anger:** People talk about the unfairness of the situation and overtly display their anger.
- **Bargaining:** This is an intermediate step when people try to correct loss by making a bargain (they will be good if loss is corrected).
- **Depression:** This is a time when people realize that this problem is really happening to them; crying, loss of appetite, and loss of energy are the usual signs.
- **Acceptance:** This is the final stage and is the acceptance of the loss.

Anticipatory grief, usually a healthy reaction, is mourning or grieving before an event has occurred (birth of a stillborn child). **Chronic grief** is mourning beyond a normal time period.

Physiological changes that occur as an individual **nears death** include the following:

- **Cardiovascular changes:** These are characterized by slowed metabolism, decreased cell oxygenation; decreased stroke volume of the heart leading to decreased ability to circulate blood effectively. The skin becomes cool, mottled, or cyanotic. Perspiration may increase because less heat is lost from the body. If dehydration is present, the temperature may rise.
- **Respiratory changes:** These are characterized by slowed or irregular breathing patterns, increased pooling of secretions in the lungs, rales, or rhonchi.
- **Neuromuscular changes:** These are characterized by severe weakness, muscle fatigue, loss of ability to swallow, loss of gag reflex, incontinence, and a decreased level of consciousness. Hearing is the last sense lost.
- **Gastrointestinal changes:** Ingestion decreases, digestion slows, constipation and ab-abdominal distension result.

Assessment of the dying patient includes the client's ability to swallow, gag reflex, circulation, respiratory function, skin for beginning signs of decubiti, comfort, stage of grief, and readiness to accept his or her impending death.

Nursing diagnoses particularly relevant to grieving include:

- Grieving, anticipatory
- Grieving, dysfunctional.

Life span concepts and death:

- **Infants and toddlers** are too young to understand death except as a loss of a caregiver.
- **Preschoolers** may experience death with the loss of a pet animal. At this age they exhibit little fear because deth seems to be only a tempoary state.
- **School-agers** begin to sense the finality of death.
- **Adolescents** and young adults feel that nothing serious can happen to them and that they will never die.
- **Middle-aged adults** recognize that death does occur, and they begin making concrete plans (will, life insurance).
- **Older adults** may think of themselves as young because they experience death with peers and relatives.

Factors influencing reactions to death:

- **Coping ability:** These include presence of support people, past successful coping mechanisms, and accurate perception of the loss or death.
- **Information available to dying persons:** This is usually given by physician. Most people appreciate knowing early that they have a terminal illness so that they can make financial and child care plans.
- **Communication blocks:** These occur when people do not know about their prognosis;

  - *Closed awareness* occurs when neither the patient nor the family knows that the patient is dying. This situation may lead to unrealistic future planning.

  - *Suspected awareness* occurs when the patient thinks that she or he is dying but lacks confirmation. The patient may lose confidence in the caregivers because the patient suspects that the caregivers are not honest.

  - *Mutual pretense awareness* occurs when the patient and the caregivers are aware of the prognosis but there is no discussion between them. The client may find it difficult to grieve, and the relationship with the caregivers may be frustrating.

Open awareness occurs when both the client and the caregivers know that the client is dying and discuss it openly in a therapeutic environment. This process facilitates planning and grieving. The presence of support people, past experiences with death, life philosophy, and the disease state influence how people will cope and accept dying and death.

Implementation of nursing care to the dying patient should focus on communication, pain, and care based on the client's changing physiological needs.

DRILL AND PRACTICE QUESTIONS FOR REVIEW

Completion Exercises

1. According to Kubler-Ross, the first stage of grieving is termed _____.

2. According to Kubler-Ross, it is the _____ stage during which the client may criticize caregivers and resist self-care.

3. According to Kubler-Ross, people need the most support during the _____ stage.

4. According to Kubler-Ross, it is the _____ stage during which clients begin to ask more questions about their illness, care, and treatment.

5. _____ is grief that extends for a very long time.

6. List three physiological changes that occur as a person nears death: _____;
_____ and _____.

7. _____ is the last sense lost as death approaches.

8. _____ grieving refers to an inability to express loss and alterations in normal sleep habits.

9. When _____ awareness occurs, neither the patient nor the family are informed that the patient is dying.

10. During _____ awareness, the patient thinks she or he is dying, but caregivers do not confirm the fact.

11. During _____ awareness, the patient, family, and caregivers discuss dying freely and openly.

12. If the patient's gag reflex is impaired, position the patient on the _____ to prevent aspiration.

13. _____ is the deliberate act of ending the life of a person suffering from an incurable, terminal, or painful disease.

14. List three advantages to dying at home: _____, _____, and _____.

15. List two disadvantages to dying at home: _____ and _____.

True/False Exercises

1. When there is a loss, a person goes through all the stags of grief outlined by Kubler-Ross.

2. Denial is a protective mechanism used to prevent people from feeling a loss.

3. According to Kubler-Ross, the first stage of grieving is the anger stage.

4. When dying patients realize that bargaining is ineffective, they usually reach a very low point in grief.

5. According to Kubler-Ross, crying and loss of appetite are usually seen during the depression stage.

6. According to Kubler-Ross, people who suffer a loss reach the acceptance stage within one year.

7. Cheyne-Stokes respirations are regular, shallow breathing patterns.

8. As people near death, there is the danger of aspiration.

9. The temperature of people nearing death, may lower because of dehydration.

10. Three factors that assist individuals toward successful coping include the presence of caring people, past successful coping patterns, and an accurate perception of loss.

11. A no-code order means that emergency measures will not be initiated if a person sustains a cardiopulmonary arrest.

12. Nurses caring for dying patients can experience the same stages of grief described by Kubler-Ross.

Situation

Mr. Green, a thirty-year-old client terminally ill with leukemia, has recently been told that his prognosis for recovery is poor. He is married and has two young children. Recently he received a grant for his research with the AIDS virus. He is angry, loud, and resistive, criticizing whatever the nurses try to do for him. As the nurse caring for him, prepare an appropriate nursing care plan.

ANSWERS TO DRILL AND PRACTICE QUESTIONS

Completion Exercises

1. denial

2. anger

3. bargaining

4. depression

5. chronic grief

6. slowed metabolism; decreased stroke volume; mottled, cool skin; dependent edema

7. hearing

8. dysfunctional

9. closed

10. suspected

11. open

12. side

13. Euthanasia

14. familiar, comforting, supportive environment; freedom from structured hospital routines; and ability to be as independent as possible

15. disruption of regular home routine; uneasiness with care needed by dying patient

True/False Exercises

1.	F		7.	F
2.	T		8.	T
3.	F		9.	F
4.	T		10.	T
5.	T		11.	T
6.	F		12.	T

The **assessment** is that Mr. Green is in the anger phase of grieving outlined by Kubler-Ross. He is expressing anger with his prognosis because he had planned on a long bright future. Believing that life is unfair, he expresses his anger in criticism and resistive behavior.

The **analysis** reveals that the client is in a grieving, anger stage that is related to his poor prognosis.

The **goal** is that the client should begin to verbalize his grief and its relationship to his self. He should move appropriately and timely through the grieving process.

The **criterion** is that the client demonstrates the ability to share his feeings with significant other (his wife).

The nursing orders should be as follows:

1. Establish and maintain a trusting relationship with the patient and his family.

2. Encourage the patient to express grief, and reassure him that his responses are normal.

3. Discuss with his wife the impact of the poor prognosis on the family unit.

4. Provide a safe, calm, comfortable, accepting, and secure environment.

5. Encourage the patient's participation in support groups.

6. Assist with ADL and decision making.

Chapter 21

UNDERSTANDING THE PERSON AS A SEXUAL BEING

NOTE TO STUDENT
The anatomy of male and female sexual organs are shown in Figure 21-2; the characteristics of normal menstrual flow are summarized in Table 21-1; and contraceptive methods are listed in Table 21-6.

MAJOR NURSING CONCEPTS

Sexuality includes sexual feelings, attitudes, and actions which are inherited and learned. Sexuality refers to a person's physical, social, emotional, intellectual, ethical thinking and behavior. **Sexual gender** (determined at the time of fertilization) refers to whether a person is male or female. **Sexual identify** is the sex a person feels and believes she or he is. **Sexual role,** which is culturally influenced, is the pattern of behavior (male or female) a person assumes. Sexual expression is manifested in dress, mannerisms, occupation, and personal touching.

The menstrual cycle is the pattern of uterine bleeding that occurs as a result of hormonal changes. **Menarche** refers to the onset of menstruation associated with puberty. **Menopause** occurs when the menstrual cycle stops for at least 1 year. The menstrual cycle involves the hypothalamus, pituitary gland, ovaries, and uterus.

- **The first phase of menstrual cycle:** The endometrium begins to increase in thickness.
- **The second phase of menstrual cycle:** The endometrium appears to be rich and spongy.
- **The ischemic phase:** when fertilization does not take place the production of progesterone and estrogen decreases. The endometrium begins to degenerate and by the twenty-fifth day sloughs off.
- **The occurrence of the menses (menstrual flow):** The flow contains approximately 25-50ml of blood, mucin, fragments of endometrial tissue, and unfertilized ovum.

Human sexual response includes excitement, plateau, orgasm, and resolution.

- **The excitement phase:** As sexual arousal occurs, the heart rate, respiratory rate, and blood pressure increase.
- **The plateau phase:** This occurs just before orgasm. The heart rate and respiratory rate increase.
- **The orgasm:** This occurs with the rhythmic contraction of genital muscles.
- **The resolution:** This is the return of male and female genital organs to the pre-excitement phase.

Peak sexual response in men usually takes place early (late teens), while the peak sexual response in women usually takes place during their late thirties.

Sexual **assessment** may be difficult because many individuals do not wish to discuss their sexual problems or concerns. It may be a subject of concern for men following surgery on their reproductive or urinary system, and for women following childbirth.

Health history and physical assessment should include information about the following: changes in weight; genital and breast development; hair distribution; hair loss from chemotherapy; inflammation, infection, or surgery on the urinary or reproductive system; spinal cord injury; coronary heart disease; and medications that may decrease sexual response, such as antihypertensives or narcotics.

Nursing diagnoses relevant to sexuality include:

- Sexual dysfunction
- Rape-trauma syndrome

Sexuality across the life span includes the following:

- Infants are cared for according to sexual gender. Girls play with dolls and wear dresses, while boys plan with sports related toys.
- Toddlers and preschoolers recognize the difference between men and women, and they begin to understand expectations of each sex role.
- School-age children become involved with activities that are androgenous.
- Adolescents establish a sense of identity and maintain a strong bond with their gender group.
- Young adults begin to express their sexuality. Middle-aged adults usually have established comfortable patterns of behavior.
- Older adults still enjoy active sexual relationships.

Mittelschmerz refers to abdominal discomfort at the time of ovulation. **Dysmenorrhea** is uncomfortable or painful menstruation. Primary dysmenorrhea occurs in the absence of disease and secondary dysmenorrhea occurs as a result of organic disease. Signs and symptoms may include bloating, cramping, pain, diarrhea, or nausea and vomiting. **Menorrhagia** is abnormally heavy menstrual flow. **Metrorrhagia** is bleeding between menstrual cycles. **Endometriosis** is the presence of uterine endometrial cells outside the uterus and may be related to excess estrogen production. **Amenorrhea** is the absence of menstrual flow and may occur because of tension, fatigue, extreme dieting, or strenuous exercise. **Toxic shock syndrome** is an infection caused by staphylococcus aureus. Signs and symptoms include fever, abdominal pain, vomiting, and diarrhea.

Sexuality problems may be the result of physical illness, obesity, disfiguring operations, trauma, erectile dysfunction, premature ejaculation, or dyspareunia (pain during coitus).

Contraceptives or birth control methods (pills, diaphragm, condoms, spermicidal creams) may decrease or interfere with sexual response. In order for **oral contraceptives** to be effective, they must be taken daily. Side effects may include nausea, weight gain, headache, and mild hypertension. Additional contraceptive methods include vaginally inserted spermicidal products; diaphragms, cervical caps, and condoms. **Natural family planning** can be accomplished by the rhythm (calendar) method, rhythm and basal temperature method, rhythm and ovulation determination, ovulation method, and coitus interruptus. Permanent methods of family planning include sterilization and vasectomy.

DRILL AND PRACTICE QUESTIONS FOR REVIEW

Completion Exercises

1. _____ refers to the cyclic uterine bleeding that occurs in females in response to hormonal changes.

2. The first menstrual period is referred to as the _____.

3. The term _____ refers to the time period during which menopausal changes take place.

4. Menopause occurs in women between _____ and _____ years.

5. The four body organs that participate in the menstrual cycle are _____, _____, _____, and _____.

6. The anterior lobe of the pituitary produces _____ and _____ which act on the ovaries and influence menses.

7. _____ suppresses hypothalamus activity.

8. _____ occurs when the ovum is released from the ovary and enters the fallopian tube.

9. Menstrual flow consists of _____, _____, and _____.

10. The four stages of sexual response are _____, _____, _____, and _____.

11. Sexually transmitted diseases are spread by _____.

12. Surgical menopause occurs with the removal of the _____ and _____.

13. Menorrhagia is _____.

14. Bleeding between menstrual cycles is termed _____.

15. Absence of menstrual flow is termed _____

16. Three methods to reduce the risk of toxic shock syndrome include _____, _____, and _____.

17. Three side effects of oral contraceptives include _____, _____, and _____.

18. Women with _____ and _____ should be carefully evaluated before being placed on contraceptive medication.

19. Diaphragms, condoms, and cervical caps are considered _____ methods of contraception.

20. Two permanent methods of family planning include _____ and _____.

True/False Exercises

1. Sexuality is biologically inherited but not culturally learned.

2. Sexual identity is the same as sexual gender.

3. Sperm carries the chromosome that determines the sex of the offspring.

4. The earlier the age of menarche, the later menopause tends to occur.

5. The goal of the menstrual cycle is to develop a mature ovum.

6. Ovulation occurs on the fourteenth day before the onset of the next menstrual cycle.

7. The body temperature of a woman rises one degree prior to the day of ovulation.

8. When fertilization does not occur, progesterone and estrogen from the ovary decrease.

9. The plateau stage of sexual response is reached after orgasm.

10. Most birth control pills contain progesterone and increase a woman's sexual response.

11. parents should be aware that masturbation is not normal for preschool boys or girls.

12. Antihypertensives and antianxiety medications diminish sexual responsiveness.

13. Men with spinal cord injuries do not have difficulty with erections or ejaculations.

14. Dysmenorrhea may be caused by the secretion of prostaglandins.

15. Aspirin is the drug of choice in the treatment of dysmenorrhea.

16. Oral contraceptives are never 100 percent safe.

17. The life of an ova is forty-eight hours.

Situation

Mary is twelve years old and has started her menses. her mother has not prepared her for this physiological and psychological change, and Mary has questions about exercise, nutrition, rest, an personal activities of daily living. List teaching points related to the above areas of concern.

ANSWERS TO DRILL AND PRACTICE QUESTIONS

Completion Exercises

1. menstrual cycle

2. menarche

3. perimenopausal

4. forty and fifty-five

5. hypothalmus, pituitary gland, ovaries, uterus

6. follicle-stimulating hormone; leuteinizing hormone

7. prolactin

8. ovulation

9. blood from ruptured capillaries, unfertilized ovum, fragments of endometrial tissue from the uterus, mucin

10. excitement, plateau, orgasm, resolution

11. coitus

12. uterus, ovaries

13. heavy menstrual flow

14. metrorrhagia

15. amenorrhea

16. use tampons made with natural fibers; change tampons often; avoid handling part of tampon that is inserted; used tampons during the day and sanitary pads at night

17. nausea, weight gain, headache, breast tenderness, spotting

18. hepatitis, diabetes, epilepsy

19. barrier

20. sterilization and vasectomy

True/False Exercises

1.	F		9.	F
2.	F		10.	F
3.	T		11.	F
4.	F		12.	T
5.	T		13.	F
6.	T		14.	T
7.	F		15.	T
8.	T		16.	F
			17.	F

Situation

Moderate exercise should be continued during menses. Excessive exercise could lead to amenorrhea. Good nutrition should be maintained; and if menstrual flow is heavy, an iron supplement may be needed. Added rest is indicated only if dysmenorrhea occurs at night, thereby interfering with needed sleep. Showering and bathing should be continued and encouraged

Chapter 22

ASSISTING THE PERSON WITH SPIRITUAL NEEDS

MAJOR NURSING CONCEPTS

An important element of holistic nursing care is assisting clients with their **spiritual needs.** Nurses should always respect their own religious beliefs.

Believing that a power higher than oneself guides life is called a **spiritual belief. Religion** refers to an organized form or worship. One's spiritual belief and religion often serve as a support system during illness. A person who denies the existence of God is called an **atheist;** an **agnostic** is a person who is uncertain about the existence of God.

When the power of God is called upon to heal instead of medical intervention, it is called **faith healing.** Nurses should support the decision to use a faith healer only when other traditional medical therapies have been exhausted. With the exception of a minor child, a person has the right to choose his or her form of therapy.

The ultimate goal of **Hinduism** is to achieve union with Brahma (God) through purity, self-control, trust, charity, compassion, and nonviolence. Hindu followers believe in reincarnation and that each person creates his or her own fate (doctrine of Karma). They may practice transcendental meditation and yoga. Hindus do not eat meat or drink alcohol.

Buddhism, which is one of the world's oldest religions, is practiced throughout Asia. Peace with God (nirvana) is the goal of life, and salvation is attained by good works. Buddhists often are vegetarians.

Many people of the Middle East and North Africa are **Islam Muslims** or **Black Muslims.** Through their sacred writings (Koran) they worship God (Allah) and study the teachings of their prophet Muhammad (not considered a savior). Black Muslims may also be dedicated to the support of black power and perpetuating black culture.

People who follow the Baha'i faith are few, but it is important for nurses to be aware of their beliefs because they must frequently fast and will rarely take medications.

Followers of **Judaism** read the Torah, are lead by a rabbi, observe their sabbath from sundown Friday to sundown Saturday, and maintain a Kosher diet. Their two most important holidays (Rosh Hashanah and Yom Kippur) occur in September or October. All male infants are circumcised on the eighth day of life. Most Orthodox Jews do not believe in postmortem examinations.

A frequently encountered form of Christianity in the United States is **Roman Catholicism.** Roman Catholics are led by a priest, read the Bible, and observe Christmas (birth of Christ) and Easter (resurrection of Christ). It is important to baptize their infants; in some instances, this may be done by the nurse. Their religious practices include communion (may take the soluble wafer even if NPO), confession, and the Sacrament of the Sick.

The **Protestant** faith has many denominations (Presbyterian, Episcopalian, Methodist, Lutheran, Baptist). Protestants are led by a minister, celebrate Christmas and Easter, and practice baptism of infants or adults, although dying without baptism is of no consequence. Most Protestants practice communion using wine or grape juice and bread, so this is not possible for the client who is NPO ("nothing-by-mouth").

Jehovah's Witnesses are another Protestant sect. Members refuse blood transfusions (in the case of a minor child, court orders may override the parent's religious wishes), feel an individual responsibility to minister to others, and rarely participate in ceremonies (Christmas, Easter, or birthday parties, for example).

The **Church of Jesus Christ of Latter-Day Saints** no longer practices polygamy. These believers highly value marriage, procreation, and parenthood. They oppose euthanasia and the use of alcohol, tea, coffee, and tobacco. The **Mennonites** and the **Amish** value simplicity and prayer. They avoid alcohol and any show of worldly wealth and gadgetry. they are excluded from social security and health insurance, and do not practice birth control.

Christian Scientists believe that healing is accomplished by prayer, not medical treatment. They often refuse medication, blood transfusions, diagnostic procedures, X-rays, surgery, and even physical examinations. Ultimately, it is the nurse's responsibility to support, inform, and respect this person's wishes and to leave the decision making to the client.

Religious beliefs help people cope with illness. A **nursing diagnoses** relevant to spiritual needs is spiritual distress (distress of the human spirit). Nurses should support their clients' religious beliefs by offering the services of hospital chaplains or offering to call the client's clergy, and by asking each client if there are any special religious activities they wish to participate in. Provide privacy for prayer and clergy visits, respect religious articles, and assist the clergy if necessary. If you are feeding a client, allow time for grace.

Unless otherwise stated, **infants** are assumed to be of the same religion as their parents. **Toddlers** have begun to formulate a sense of right and wrong, and **preschoolers** have an elemental concept of a God. Young hospitalized children are comforted by religious traditions such as grace before meals, bedtime prayers, and celebrating religious holidays. Because **school-agers** are rule-oriented, they expect that God practices the rule that good behavior reaps good rewards. An ill child of this age may feel illness is a form of punishment. **Adolescents** frequently question the existence of God and may shun religious practices. The **young adult** and **middle-aged adult** may reincorporate religion into their lifestyles. Conflict can arise when a marriage has merged two religious beliefs. Adults especially enjoy their religious celebrations. There is the tendency for **older adults** to increase their religiosity.

DRILL AND PRACTICE QUESTIONS FOR REVIEW

Complete the statements below.

1. One who does not believe in the existence of a God is called a/an _____.

2. _____ is any form of organized worship.

3. An exercise practiced by Hindus to attain bodily and mental well-being is called _____.

4. When caring for a Hindu patient, the nurse may have to determine whether or not this patient's medications contain _____.

5. Many Buddhists eat a _____ diet.

6. _____ and _____ are prohibited in the Muslim's diet.

7. Most Orthodox Jews maintain a _____ diet.

8. When a Roman Catholic is hospitalized, it would be appropriate for the nurse to notify the hospital priest, who may perform a rite called _____.

9. Two Protestant denominations which denounce the use of blood transfusions are _____ and _____.

10. The age group most likely to avoid religious observations is _____.

Determine whether the following statements are TRUE or FALSE.

1. Having a spiritual belief means the person is committed to an organized form of worship.

2. Religion influences emotional and physical health.

3. Healing by the power of God instead of by medical treatments is referred to as faith healing.

4. Repeated chanting is a form of prayer used by Hindus.

5. Muslims believe in reincarnation.

6. It is not necessary for the nurse to observe an infant following a religious circumcision.

7. In an emergency, the nurse may baptize a Roman Catholic infant by pouring water on the head and saying, "I baptize you in the name of the Father, and of the Son, and the Holy Spirit."

8. It is important for nurses to make decisions for their clients when there is a conflict between medical and religious practices.

9. Holy oil which has been applied to the body of a Roman Catholic client should be allowed to dry naturally.

10. Members of the Church of Jesus Christ of Latter-Day Saints will not consume coffee, tea, alcohol, or tobacco.

Situations

Situation 1

Johnny Moore is a nine-year-old admitted to the hospital for an appendectomy (surgical removal of the appendix). His mother is at his bedside. List specific nursing considerations you would incorporate into your care plan for Johnny which are pertinent to his Roman Catholic religious background.

Situation 2

Mr. Cohen is a 60 year old Orthodox Jew with a two-month history of abdominal pain. He is admitted to the hospital for diagnostic tests and has a tentative diagnosis of "rule out cancer of the colon." List specific nursing considerations you would incorporate into your care plan for Mr. Cohen which are pertinent to his Jewish religious background.

ANSWERS TO DRILL AND PRACTICE QUESTIONS

Completion Exercises

1. atheist
2. Religion
3. yoga
4. alcohol
5. vegetarian
6. Pork, alcohol
7. kosher
8. the Sacrament of the Sick
9. Jehovah's Witnesses, Christian Scientist
10. adolescents

True/False Exercises

1. F
2. T
3. T
4. T
5. F

6. F
7. T
8. F
9. T
10. T

Situations

Situation 1

- Ask Mrs. Moore the specific prayers Johnny usually says before meals and at bedtime.
- Ask the hospital priest or Johnny's priest to visit Johnny and his mother.
- Provide privacy during clergy visits.
- Respect and treat carefully any religious objects at the bedside such as rosaries.
- Allow this school-ager time to verbalize his feelings about why God allowed him to become ill.

Situation 2

- Arrange for a kosher diet.
- Consult with Mr. Cohen's physician in order to avoid elective procedures on Mr. Cohen's sabbath (Saturday).
- Encourage visits by his rabbi.
- Provide privacy during clergy visits and during prayer time.
- Respect religious articles such as prayer shawls and books.

Chapter 23

PROMOTION OF INDIVIDUAL, FAMILY, AND COMMUNITY HEALTH

MAJOR NURSING CONCEPTS

Nurses work in a variety of settings, including schools, industry, clinics, hospitals, and homes. Nurses working in the community assist in maintaining individual, family, and community health. This area of nursing is chiefly concerned with prevention of illness and restoration of health.

Areas of care:

- direct or individual care: given to people discharged from health care agencies, who are still in need of assistance and nursing care (wound dressings)

- family care: nurses assist family members in adjusting to health problem (nutrition)

- community care: focus is on information people about potential health dangers (pollution)

Individuality refers to characteristics that make a person unique. They include maturity, intelligence, education, position in the family, temperament, level of health, sex, past experience, environment, education, and life style.

- maturity: refers to judgment and reasoning ability

- intelligence: people with low-level intelligence may have difficulty learning health-care techniques

- education level: influences problem-solving abilities

- ordinal position in family: first-born children may have more restrictions on behavior; younger children may be more skilled at problem solving; middle children may feel insecure

- temperament: refers to traits and behavioral responses to various situations. According to Thomas and Chess (1977) the following are patterns of temperament:

  - activity level: includes energy level, motor activity

  - rhythmicity: refers to cyclic patterns of behavior

  - approach: initial response to a new situation

  - adaptability: ability to alter responses to events

  - intensity of reaction: may include overreaction to situations

  - distractibility: ability to shift to different activities

  - attention span and persistence: varies with individuals

  - threshold of responsiveness: refers to the intensity of the stimuli necessary to elicit a response

- mood quality: overall tone of feelings in response to others (happy, sad, complaining)
- level of health: state of health can influence ability to adapt to events
- past experiences: past responses may influence current behavior
- environment: reactions to situations may differ according to setting
- life style: manner in which people behave is related to their behavioral characteristics

Role of Support People:

- first level: individuals who live close to the client or have strong emotional ties to client, usually family members or significant others
- second level: includes friends, neighbors, and distant relatives
- third level: includes individuals in the workplace, school, or community associations
- fourth level: refers to the world population

A **family** may be defined as a group of people living together for their mutual benefit, who have shared mutual interests. Types of families include the following:

- nuclear family: usually composed of husband, wife, and children
- extended family: includes nuclear family, grandparents, aunts, uncles, cousins, and grand-children
- single-parent family: refers to only one parent living at home
- single-adult family
- communal family: comprises groups of people living together as an extended family group; relationship is based on social-values or interests
- cohabitation families: refers to unmarried couples living together
- homosexual unions: includes persons of the same sex living together as a married couple

According to **Duvall,** families pass through the following stages:

- marriage: members learn how to handle finances, relatives, sex, and daily household routines
- early childbearing: both partners learn to accept the responsibility of child care
- families with preschool children: parents adjust to busy family-life events and strengthen family unity
- families with school-age children: parents prepare children for future responsibilities and increase their own earning power
- families with adolescent children: parents loosen family ties so that their children can learn to be independent
- launching center families: children leave home, partners return to a two-member family
- families of middle years: two-member family is complete
- family in retirement or old age: may consist of one member

Family assessment includes identifying and contacting family members who will assume responsibility for client care.

Community assessment includes knowledge of the following:

- housing system: heat, water supply, housing repairs

- transportation system: client's ability to visit health-care facilities for follow-up care

- education system: access to centers in order to learn new skills

- age-span system: young community will provide needed health-care services for the frequent illnesses of childhood; communities with mostly aged adults will have few resources for young parents

- sociocultural system: values, beliefs, and life styles influence health care, health education, and level of health

- financial occupational system: work influences health, financial status, housing, education, and recreation system

- political system: influences monies spent on health-care facilities and education

- recreational system: communities differ as to recreational opportunities available; recreational facilities reflect communities' value of recreation

- safety-protection system: includes fire, law enforcement, sanitation, and water supply

- religious system: religious beliefs and values influence religious activities and facilities available for worship

- environmental system: includes air pollution, water supply, and psychological feelings of the community

- health-care system: community concerns differ as to preventive vs. restorative care as well as to availability and access to health care

DRILL AND PRACTICE QUESTIONS FOR REVIEW

Completion Exercises

1. Nurses are employed in community settings such as _____, _____, and _____.

2. Areas of care for community health nurses include the _____, _____, and _____.

3. Community health nurses are concerned with _____, _____, and _____.

4. Three characteristics that differentiate people and make them unique include _____, _____, and _____.

5. _____ children may develop behavior problems as they grow and develop because they did not die as expected.

6. Three patterns of temperament identified by Thomas and Chess are _____, _____, and _____.

7. The first level of support people include _____ and _____.

8. A family may be defined as a _____.

9. Duvall states that the first stage of family development is _____.

10. A family assessment should include information on _____ and _____ .

11. An assessment of client needs based on characteristics of individuality should include information on _____ and _____ .

True/False Exercises

1. Community health nurses do not participate in secondary level of prevention.

2. Nurses may not administer medications in the home.

3. Maturity refers to a person's ability to reason and problem-solve.

4. A client under stress may be expected to lose his or her problem-solving and decision-making abilities.

5. All children in the same family will grow up with the same thinking and problem-solving abilities.

6. Degrees of persistence and attention span (Thomas and Chess) vary slightly.

7. According to Thomas and Chess, approach refers to a person's response to a new and unfamiliar situation.

8. According to Thomas and Chess, mood quality refers to overall tone of feelings in response to others.

9. Nursing-care planning should be the same for all patients with similar problems.

10. The second level of support people include the client's friends, neighbors, and relatives outside the immediate family.

11. The fourth level of support people include individuals in the client's community or workplace.

12. A community assessment includes information about a client's housing, transportation, and education system.

13. Health-care availability is similar from community to community.

Situation

Mr. Kramer is a sixty-two-year-old married man who is going to be discharged from the hospital in two days. He lives in a one-family house with his wife; his daughter lives nearby. Mr. Kramer has had extensive abdominal surgery and will be on oral antibiotics for ten more days. Mr. Kramer ambulates slowly and needs assistance with bathing, dressing, and toileting. Mrs. Kramer is fifty-seven years old and has been taught how to care for his wound. Mr. Kramer is scheduled for a follow-up visit with his physician in two weeks. Prepare a nursing care plan for discharge.

ANSWERS TO DRILL AND PRACTICE QUESTIONS

Completion Exercises

1. schools, industry, clinics, hospitals, and homes

2. individual, family, and community

3. water/environmental pollution, availability of and access to health-care facilities, physical and psychological needs of dying patients and their families

4. intelligence, maturity, temperament, sex, state of health, past experience, education level, and life style

5. vulnerable

6. activity level, rhythmicity, approach, adaptability, intensity of reaction, distractibility, attention span, responsiveness, and mood

7. family members, people with strong emotional ties

8. group of individuals sharing the same living arrangements for shared mutual interests

9. marriage

10. decision maker, nurturer, problem solver, finances, safety, and state of health

11. maturity, intelligence, education level, special needs pertaining to temperament, environment, life style, and level of health

True/False Exercises

1.	F	7.	T
2.	F	8.	T
3.	T	9.	F
4.	T	10.	T
5.	F	11	F
6.	F	12.	T
		13.	F

Situation

Assessment

- Physical status: Client needs assistance with bathing, grooming, toileting, ambulation, and wound care.
- Housing: Client lives in a one-family house that has ample heat, electricity, plumbing, and water.
- Type of family: The family are of middle years.
- Family characteristics: Wife is active, knowledgeable, and willing to help her husband with his needs; daughter lives close by.
- Dominant family figure: Both partners share in problem solving and decision making.
- Finances: Medical bills are covered by insurance; Mrs. Kramer works part-time as a salesperson; Mr. Kramer is an accountant; there are adequate income and savings.
- Home safety: The home is safe, well-lighted, and uncluttered; there is ample room for Mrs. Kramer to assist her husband in ambulation so that falls should not occur; both have good vision.

- Health care: Client has a private physician and has telephone number if he should have questions.
- Religious affiliation: Both partners attend church weekly, and daughter will transport.

Nursing diagnosis:

Self care deficit (bathing, dressing, toileting, and ambulation) related to surgery and early hospital discharge.

Goal:

Mr. Kramer should be able to perform self-care activities within his level of ability post discharge.

Criteria:

Mr. Kramer eagerly, safely, and independently performs self-care activities of bathing, grooming, toileting, and ambulation.

Nursing Orders:
- Review importance of returning to physician for follow-up care.
- Review physician's prescriptions for medication, activity, and wound care.
- Review principles of cleanliness and good hygiene to help prevent a wound infection.
- Review principles of safe transfer and ambulation to prevent falls.
- Advise couple on proper nutrition.
- Promote patient participation in performing activities of daily living.
- Inform wife that she should allow sufficient time for patient to complete activities.

Chapter 24

PROVIDING NURSING CARE IN THE HOME

MAJOR NURSING CONCEPTS

Home health care involves the delivery of comprehensive health-care services (health promotion, disease prevention, illness and rehabilitative care) to patients in their homes. Reimbursement constraints imposed by DRG's (Diagnostic-Related Groups) have caused hospitals to discharge patients more quickly, increasing the number of patients requiring care in the home. Sophisticated treatments have recently become feasible in the home setting, and patients prefer to be cared for in their own home.

The nurse who provides care in the home may be an independent practitioner or an employee of a **home health-care agency** (certified or licensed to provide services that are reimbursable by Medicare/Medicaid) or of a **home health-care service** (private corporation). A nurse may also function in home care as an employee of a **hospice** (facility that provides care for the terminally ill) or a specialized service, such as one that provides for the administration of IV antibiotic therapy.

Both **direct services** (nursing assessments and actions) and **indirect services** (case-finding, collaboration with and/or referral to other health-care providers, family assessment/intervention, supervision of care) are provided. **Skilled nursing care** (physician-ordered treatments or procedures) is reimbursable by Medicare/Medicaid and by many private insurers. Physician-ordered services provided by **home health aides** (trained to provide personal care, simple tasks, and monitor vital signs), **homemakers** (trained to provide assistance with activities of daily living), and therapists are also reimbursable by Medicare/Medicaid, but generally not by private insurers.

Nurses are involved in assessing the quality of services provided by home health-care agencies or services. Certified or licensed agencies meet predetermined standards for the delivery of quality care. Agencies that provide high-quality care generally have a code of ethics, publish policies and procedures, and provide for staff education.

Patients in need of home care services include the elderly; those who have need for assistance with ADL; those requiring sophisticated treatments (IV therapy, ostomy care, oxygen therapy, terminal illness care, wound care/dressings); and those requiring assessment and intervention (i.e., teaching) to help them deal with a chronic health problem or life style change. For home health care to be successful, the patient must have a support system in the home. A **care partner** may assume the role of caregiver in the absence of the nurse. Collaboration between the nurse who cared for a patient in an in-patient setting and the home health care nurse is essential to the success of home health care.

When caring for a patient in his or her home, the environment should be assessed for **safety** to determine whether home management of care is feasible and safe. Assessment may be a challenge, and **distractors in the environment** need to be limited so that assessment can be accomplished. When planning care in the home, goals should be mutually agreed upon by the nurse and the patient. The home health care nurse may have to **adapt and improvise** in the administration of care and procedures in the home. The nursing care provided should be comprehensive and aimed at meeting total patient care needs, not just those that are reimbursable by an insurer. Education is an essential component of home health care. Patients and/or caregivers must know when and how to obtain direction or help if necessary. Documentation of care should be clear, specific, and comprehensive so that reimbursement, if entitled, can occur.

DRILL AND PRACTICE QUESTIONS FOR REVIEW

Complete the statements below.

1. For nursing services to be reimbursable under Medicare/Medicaid regulations, those services must be physician-ordered treatments or procedures. These constitute _____ nursing care.

2. A nonnurse health-care provider who is trained to provide personal care and to monitor vital signs is called a _____.

3. A private company that provides for the delivery of home care services is called a home health-care _____.

4. A support person who is willing to assume the role of caregiver in the home is called a _____.

5. A nurse assesses that a patient's caregiver is becoming physically exhausted. In this situation, it would be appropriate to investigate whether or not _____ care is available in the community.

6. Despite adequate support systems, a patient's home environment continues to be unsafe for provision of health care. An appropriate nursing diagnosis would be _____.

7. Terminally ill patients requiring counseling and/or other services in the home can be referred to a community-based _____ to determine what services are available.

8. A community-based service that provides meals for home-bound persons is called _____.

Determine whether the following statements are TRUE or FALSE.

1. Because of constraints imposed by the home environment, it is not feasible to provide comprehensive care in the home.

2. Under the DRG system, patients are discharged from hospitals with increased need for nursing services in the home.

3. Nurses recently licensed to practice nursing are ideal candidates for employment in home health-care settings.

4. It is important that procedures be carried out exactly the same in both in-patient settings and the home environment so that patients do not become confused.

5. A nurse is caring for a patient in a home setting that is very different from her own. She should acknowledge that the quality of her nursing care will suffer and request not to care for this patient again.

6. Documentation of care is especially important for care provided in home-care settings to insure that reimbursement is obtained for provided services.

Classify each of the activities specified below as a DIRECT or an INDIRECT nursing service.

1. The nurse assesses that a patient requires the services of a podiatrist. He or she appropriately refers the patient.

2. The nurse performs a wound irrigation and a dressing change.

3. The nurse teaches a patient self-administration of insulin.

4. The nurse administers a patient's medication.

5. The nurse assesses the patient's family situation and determines eligibility and need for public assistance.

6. The nurse supervises care provided by a home health aide.

Situation

You are a nurse working for a home health-care agency. You will provide care today for 62-year-old Jim Johnson. This is his first visit from a home health care nurse. Yesterday he was discharged from the hospital with an abdominal wound that requires a daily wound irrigation and dressing change. State the assessments that you will carry out in this first home-care visit.

ANSWERS TO DRILL AND PRACTICE QUESTIONS

Completion Exercises

1. skilled
2. home health aide
3. service
4. care partner
5. respite
6. Home maintenance management: Impaired
7. hospice
8. Meals-on-Wheels

True/False Exercises

1. F
2. T
3. F
4. F
5. F
6. T

Classify the Activity

1. indirect
2. direct
3. direct
4. direct
5. indirect
6. indirect

Situation

   Assessment:

   - support people in the home
   - ability of patient-support persons to assess wound for signs and symptoms that suggest need for immediate medical intervention and obtain help as necessary
   - ability of patient to perform ADL
   - safety of the environment
   - patient's eligibility for insurance reimbursement of services and/or other means of payment
   - patient knowledge of wound care/dressing change procedure

PART VI

THE NURSE AS AN EFFECTIVE COMMUNICATOR

Chapter 25

THERAPEUTIC COMMUNICATION

NOTE TO STUDENT

Focus on Nursing Care outlines ten principles for good listening and is located at the end of this chapter.

MAJOR NURSING CONCEPTS

Communication is defined as a verbal or nonverbal exchange of ideas between two or more individuals. It is an important active process that is integral to the nurse-client relationship. Communication can be divided into two categories: nontherapeutic (social, everyday conversation) and therapeutic (helpful, goal-oriented). **Nontherapeutic communication** lacks structure, planning, or purpose other than casual conversation; it does not attempt to change behavior. **Therapeutic communication** has structure and is planned to be helpful and change behavior. It requires practice and concentration, and is the essence of a therapeutic, helping nurse-client relationship.

Communication components consist of the encoder, code, decoder, and response, or feedback, loop. The **encoder** refers to the person who originates the message. The **code** is the verbal or nonverbal message, thought, or feeling that is transmitted. Various methods include poems, novels, computers, paintings, radio, and television. With the **decoder,** the receiver of the message decodes or interprets the message (cognitive processing). People interpret messages in different ways, based on past knowledge and experience.

The **feedback/response loop** refers to the reply that the receiver of the message (decoder) returns to the sender. This reply could be verbal or nonverbal (touch, nod, facial grimace). With the reply, the receiver has become the sender of a message. Feedback informs people whether or not their message was understood.

Communication patterns differ across the life span.

1. In the **infant,** response is shown with total body movement—kicks, cries, and thrashing arms. By eight weeks of age, spontaneous communication of a "dovelike, cooing" sound occurs; smiling becomes apparent, and the infant is fun to be with. Crying can be differentiated (hunger, pain), and parents can interpret messages more accurately. At six months, infants can usually utter repetitively discernable sounds ("oh, da"), and by nine months "da-da" is audible.

2. The **toddler** acquires new words and learns simple word structure. Also, the toddler begins to encode verbal messages; the vocabulary may consist of approximately one thousand words.

3. The **preschooler** asks many questions, using language in order to find answers to his or her world. In addition, the preschooler learns words that have more than one meaning.

4. The **school-age child** learns to read and to operate a computer. Verbal language becomes expressive; the level of language development and usage reflects family life and environment.

5. The **adolescent** uses a small part of his or her total learned vocabulary and also often uses slang words and words with sexual connotations because such usage helps identify adolescents with their peers and helps to achieve a strong sense of personal identity.

6. In the **adult,** communication patterns vary greatly, depending on culture, education level, and work situation.

7. The **older adult** may demonstrate a slower pattern of speech or an inability to give feedback. **Aphasia** may be defined as a sensory or motor disorder that affects the comprehension of language; it is the inability to understand or use verbal or nonverbal communication. **Dysarthria** refers to difficulties with language articulation or expression.

Levels of communication vary, and according to **Powell** (1969), may be categorized in five levels.

The **first level, cliché conversation,** refers to pleasant greetings such as "have a nice day" and "how are you." These clichés reflect a superficial relationship and are used often at the outset of a new relationship. The **second level, fact reporting,** implies stating facts about yourself that help others know who you are, such as information about your age, occupation, or medical problem. At the **third level, shared personal ideas and judgments** the beginning level of a therapeutic interaction is formed. At the **fourth level, shared feelings** feelings are communicated only if trust is established. Reaching the **fifth level, peak communication,** implies a type of communication that reflects total understanding of the other person; this understanding arises out of a long-standing relationship between caring, trusting individuals.

Nonverbal communication is considered as important as verbal communication and may be expressed in the following ways:

The **use of distance** is culturally influenced and reflects personal experience. Intimate space, which is the space directly surrounding an individual, is up to a distance of 18 inches from the body (bathing a patient). Personal space is from 18 inches to 4 feet (talking on the telephone). Social space is the distance between 4 feet and 12 feet (classroom teaching). Public space is the distance beyond 12 feet and requires shouting.

The **feeling of genuineness** is a sincere, honest quality of being yourself. It forms the basis for a trusting, therapeutic relationship.

The **feeling of warmth** is a quality that is demonstrated by a gentle tone of voice, attentive listening, direct eye contact, and respecting a person's intimate an personal space. It arises after you know a person well.

The **feeling of empathy** is the ability to place yourself in another person's situation and to experience that person's feelings. Empathetic individuals serve as the best support people because they can anticipate another person's reaction to a new and stressful situation.

The **use of gestures** is culturally influenced and reflects individual characteristics. If gestures are not used correctly, they may be misinterpreted.

Body posture and gait reflect one's mental state. People with good self-esteem usually have an upright body posture and walk rapidly with assurance and confidence. People who are depressed tend to slouch and walk slowly without determination or boldness.

General appearance, especially clothes, may reflect the self-esteem of the encoder and the intensity and importance of the person's message.

The **use of touch** is an intimate, meaningful method of nonverbal communication, which needs to be used carefully because of cultural variation and individual preferences.

The **use of humor** is important, since people who have the ability to laugh at their own mistakes are usually good company. Humor must be used discriminately and evaluated carefully with the ill client.

Using drawings is a way to identify and understand a potentially frightening experience for a child. A child's use of colors (crayons) may also assist health-care professionals in identifying depression or low self-esteem.

The **use of music** help identify the mood people are in and how they feel about themselves.

There are several techniques that facilitate **therapeutic communication.** The first is **attentive listening** followed by **questioning. Open-ended questions** allow a person the latitude to answer in a variety of responses; direct questions limit responses because they require a simple answer to a specific question. **Reflecting** is the technique of restating the last word or phrase that the person has said. This technique makes the encoder feel that you are attentively and actively listening to the message. **Clarifying** consists of repeating ideas that people have stated in order to assure understanding of the message. **Paraphrasing** consists of changing the person's exact words while retaining the meaning of the words. **Perception checking** consists of validating a feeling or emotion that is stated. **Focusing** is a technique that includes repeating a statement or mentioning an avoided topic. This technique helps a person focus on a difficult subject in order to begin to solve a problem. **Supportive statements** inform the clients that you accept their behavior. **Silence** allows the client time to think and offer more information than originally asked for.

Factors that may **interfere** with effective communication include age and developmental level, intellectual level, physical factors (pain, hearing, and speech defects), emotional factors (anxiety or grief), social factors (culture or ethnic background), and environmental factors (extreme temperatures, excessive noises).

Blocks to effective communication include changing the subject, offering false reassurance, offering one's personal opinion, telling people how they should feel, using technical terminology, inattentive listening, showing disapproval, not showing approval, being defensive, and giving personal advice.

Special communication skills are required with the shy, angry demanding, or sexually aggressive client because of insecurity, fear, and frustration. The client with a language barrier, the unconscious client, and the client with vision or hearing impairment also have special needs requiring specific communication skills.

A **Nursing diagnosis** pertinent would be:

- Communication, impaired verbal.

The nurse-patient relationship is built on trust and rapport. It develops through several phases. In the **initiation phase,** introductions are made, and many questions are asked in order to learn valuable basic, needed information. The initiation may last for a few minutes; sincerity and honesty are basic to this phase of the nurse-patient relationship. The **working phase** consists of working actively with clients toward completing the task of maintaining or restoring their health. The **termination phase** is the time for the nurse-patient relationship to end; usually goals have been reached and patients can do more for themselves. It is important for the nurse to recognize clients who are unable to care for themselves so that appropriate planning can take place.

DRILL AND PRACTICE QUESTIONS FOR REVIEW

Complete the statements below.

1. Communication can best be described as an _____.

2. Nontherapeutic communication can be identified by its _____ and _____.

3. Therapeutic communication can be identified by _____ and _____.

4. The communication process consists of the following components: _____, _____, _____, and _____.

5. In addition to verbal communication _____, _____, and _____ are additional ways people communicate.

6. Cognitive processing refers to _____.

7. Ineffective communication may be the result of _____.

8. Infants respond to their new environment by _____.

9. Older adults may have difficulty with speech because _____.

10. The five levels of communication are _____, _____, _____, _____, and _____.

11. The use of distance is affected by _____ and _____.

12. Social distance is the space between _____ and _____.

13. _____ is the quality of being yourself.

14. _____ is the ability to understand what another person is feeling and experiencing.

15. The use of touch is affected by _____ and _____.

16. Three techniques that encourage therapeutic communication are _____, _____, and _____.

17. _____ consists of repeating ideas in order to avoid vague, incomplete statements.

18. Three factors that interfere with effective communication are _____, _____, and _____.

19. Two specific blocks to effective communication are _____ and _____.

20. _____ and _____ are two techniques that can be used to effect good listening.

True/False Exercises

1. Nontherapeutic communication consists of social, everyday conversation.

2. Nonverbal communication is not considered therapeutic communication.

3. The encoder is the person who begins the interaction.

4. Communication can still be effective if cognitive processing does not take place.

5. Messages may be misinterpreted if the receiver has a different education level or misses part of the message.

6. People under stress may have difficulty understanding messages.

7. Feedback tells the encoder that the message has been received and interpreted accurately.

8. Toddlers acquire many new words and begin to put together short phrases.

9. School-age children can learn to use a computer at age eight.

10. Language reflects education level, culture, and work environment.

11. Aphasia may refer to difficulties with expressions of sound.

12. Intimate space may be defined as the distance up to 18 inches from the body.

13. A sense of oneness is achieved in the fifth level of communication.

14. Reflecting involves restating what has been verbally or nonverbally communicated.

15. Silence is a technique that encourages therapeutic communication.

16. Although touch communicates caring, it is inappropriate to use with clients.

Situation

Mr. Gold is a seventy-year-old patient hospitalized because of a cerebral vascular accident (stroke). He has difficulty finding the appropriate words, articulating words, and identifying objects. In addition, he easily becomes anxious, frustrated, and angry. As the nurse caring for this patient, list five appropriate nursing actions with rationale.

ANSWERS TO DRILL AND PRACTICE QUESTIONS

Completion Exercises

1. exchange of ideas or feelings between two or more people

2. lack of structure, planning, or purpose

3. structure, planning and goal orientation

4. encoder, code, decoder, and feedback or response

5. drawings, television, touching, paintings, and computers

6. interpretation of message

7. no feedback, feedback given before message was understood, or misinterpretation of message

8. total body involvement to stimuli, i.e., kicking, thrashing

9. physiological changes in the brain or neurological involvement

10. cliché, fact reporting, shared personal ideas, shared feelings, and peak communication
11. culture and personal preference
12. 4 feet and 12 feet
13. genuineness
14. empathy
15. culture and personal preference
16. effective, attentive listening, open-ended questions, reflecting, clarifying, and paraphrasing
17. clarifying
18. age, intellectual level, physical, social or environmental factors
19. changing the subject, offering false reassurance, and giving opinions and advice
20. stop talking, make people comfortable, remove distractions, be patient and at ease, and ask questions

True/False Exercises

1.	T	9.	T
2.	F	10.	T
3.	T	11.	T
4.	F	12.	T
5.	T	13.	T
6.	T	14.	T
7.	T	15.	T
8.	T	16.	F

Situation

Nursing actions and rationale:

1. Determine languages understood and spoken; determine cultural background and personal preferences related to touch and distance. In order for messages to be understood, they need to be in the language that the client understands. Cultural background and individual preferences are the basis for determining the use of touch and the appropriate distance for therapeutic communication to occur.

2. Observe, listen, and determine the meaning of Mr. Gold's verbal and nonverbal expressions. This approach will prevent misinterpretation.

3. Maintain a calm, patient, unhurried manner. This approach will allow enough time for Mr. Gold to communicate, and it should help to reduce his frustration and anger.

4. Visit the patient often; anticipate his needs and ask questions that require short answers. This approach should help to decrease frustration and anger.

5. Decrease environmental stimuli so that Mr. Gold can concentrate on efforts to communicate. This approach will also help to reduce frustration and anxiety.

6. Elicit the aid of a speech pathologist.

7. Include family members in the care. This approach will help the family understand, accept, provide support, and develop the necessary skills required at this time.

Chapter 26

DOCUMENTATION OF NURSING CARE

NOTE TO STUDENT

Guidelines for documenting nursing care are listed in Table 1; examples of narrative and problem oriented-recording are described at the end of the chapter.

MAJOR NURSING CONCEPTS

Client records are legal documentation of care and are confidential. There are a number of reasons for keeping client records:

- **Aid to diagnosis:** The data base is recorded and serves as a guide toward diagnosis.
- **Continuity and justification of care:** The record aids in determining if therapies are successful.
- **Communication between health care personnel:** Health-care providers can discover what other personnel have prescribed, thereby preventing duplication and inadequate care.
- **Legal documentation of care:** Records are required by law and accrediting agencies. They may be used as evidence in court.
- **Research:** Records serve as data base for statistics. They may also serve as a base for determining community health-care needs.
- **Education:** Records are used as a source for teaching and learning.
- **Quality assurance audit:** This audit is required by state, federal, and hospital accrediting agencies. Charts are reviewed to determine quality of care, using predetermined standards of care.
- **Documentation for DRGs:** In order for agencies to receive payment for services (according to Diagnostic Related Groups), care must be documented.
- **Individualization of care:** Records facilitate personalized nursing-care plans.

Types of client records include the following:

- The **information (personal data/admission) sheet** lists basic, necessary information such as the client's name, address, birth date, religion, occupation, physician, insurance coverage, date of hospitalization, and diagnosis.
- The **face (graphic) sheet** provides a quick reference for vital signs (TPR B/P), and intake and output.
- The **physician's order sheet** contains all orders/treatments.
- The **client's history sheet** lists health history and findings from the physical examination.

114

- The **physician's progress sheet** is used to describe progress and response to therapies.
- The laboratory and diagnostic findings forms
- The **nursing progress notes** contain **narrative charting** written in **chronological order.** They include an assessment of physical and psychosocial factors, an assessment of the client's environment; a documentation of care; a response of the client to care; a documentation of care done by others; a documentation of visitors including clergy; and educational information given to client/family. Also the nursing progress notes contain **problem-oriented recording,** in which information is categorized and documented according to the client's problems rather than when events occurred.
- **Additional forms** include medication records, flow sheets, and consent forms.

Nursing Kardex is a quick, easy, client record-keeping system.

DRILL AND PRACTICE QUESTIONS FOR REVIEW

Completion Exercises

1. Three purposes for maintaining client records are _____, _____, and _____.

2. _____ audit is required by the Joint Commission of Accreditation of Hospitals.

3. Client records generally consist of _____, _____, and _____ forms.

4. _____ forms grant permission for health care.

5. Narrative charting should include _____, _____, and _____.

6. A discharge note should include _____, _____, and _____.

7. _____ recording is done according to client problems rather than sequence of events.

8. Information that is told to you by the client and cannot be observed is termed _____ data.

True/False Exercises

1. Accurate documentation should prevent inadequate care.

2. Client records contain legal and confidential information.

3. Clients have access to their medical record in all states.

4. Quality assurance audits help identify client care problems.

5. Nursing care should be documented before care is administered.

6. Professional nurses are required to understand laboratory studies.

7. Informed consent is necessary for procedures that involve special risk to the client.

8. Pain is considered objective data.

9. When documenting care on a progress sheet, blank lines should be left between recordings.

10. Errors in recording should be erased.

ANSWERS TO DRILL AND PRACTICE QUESTIONS

Completion Exercises

1. continuity of care, communication, research, teaching
2. quality assurance
3. information sheet, face sheet, physician's order form, history, progress sheet, consent form, and medication sheet
4. consent
5. physiological and psychological factors, procedures, client's response to care, teaching
6. time, method, medications, equipment, client's appearance, follow-up care
7. problem-oriented
8. subjective

True/False Exercises

1.	T	6.	Y
2.	T	7.	T
3.	F	8.	F
4.	T	9.	F
5.	F	10.	F

Chapter 27

CLIENT TEACHING

MAJOR NURSING CONCEPTS

Client teaching is a primary nursing responsibility and may be done in a **group** situation or on an **individual** basis, **informally** or **formally.**

Principles of good teaching include the following: (1) **knowing the subject** means being thoroughly knowledgeable about the subject you are teaching; (2) **knowing your learning audience** refers to using teaching methods appropriate to developmental needs and interests of the clients; (3) **knowing yourself** is the ability to identify the teaching strategies you are most comfortable using; (4) **expressing individual learning styles** includes establishing a rapport with the learner in order to determine which teaching technique is most effective in the given situation; (5) **defining teaching goals** allows the nurse to identify the specific parts of a subject pertinent to the individual client or group; (6) **providing an environment and time conducive to learning** is choosing to teach under the best circumstances with the least number of distractions; (7) **being consistent** means teaching a skill only one way in order to avoid confusion; (8) recognizing the effectiveness of **nonverbal teaching** refers to avoiding contradiction in your verbal and nonverbal messages; (9) **teaching principles** is teaching someone why he or she is doing something, thus giving the person the ability to modify actions in different situations; (10) **teaching what people should do, not what they should not** makes learning more enjoyable by providing a positive viewpoint; (11) **being specific** means giving explicit and clear information; (12) **teaching from the simple to the complex** is beginning with basic knowledge and slowly moving to more complex material; (13) **acknowledging that people may learn more than you teach** allows for the learner to continue the learning process by expanding on what he or she has learned; and (14) **including evaluation** determines the effectiveness of your teaching.

Cognitive learning refers to a change in a person's understanding of knowledge. **Psychomotor learning** is acquiring the ability to perform a motor skill. **Affective learning** involves an attitude change.

Nurses, as client teachers, needs to know that learning occurs only **when a person is ready to learn;** that it occurs most quickly if the **person understands the importance of the information;** and that it occurs best if **rewards,** not penalties, **are offered.** People learn best by **actively participating** in learning in a nonstressful and **accepting environment.** People also learn best those things that **hold a particular interest** for them; and even then, people reach a point of saturation **(learning ability plateaus),** and learning temporarily stops.

Teaching techniques vary according to the developmental learning abilities of people throughout the lifespan. A teaching strategy appropriate for an **infant** is game playing; for the **toddler** it is playing "Simon Says"; for the **preschooler,** use short explanations and demonstrations; and for the **schoolage child,** use participation in projects. **Adolescents** like to learn things separate from their parents, and teaching strategies should not emphasize future benefits but should emphasize more immediate rewards. Teaching strategies for the **young adult, middle-aged adult,** and **older adult** should include the importance of the learning so that they may continue to live independently and should also include significant others as support persons.

117

Developing a **teaching plan** involves several preliminary **steps.** First, **assess the client's current knowledge** in order not to under teach or over teach. Second, **assess the client's physical capabilities** in order to determine whether the client is able to perform the psycho-motor skill you plan to teach. Third, **assess the client's psychological or emotional capabilities,** because people have more difficulty learning if they have a low self-esteem or if they find the topic distasteful. Fourth, **be aware of the client's attention span** so you can alter your teaching strategies accordingly. Fifth, **ascertain** the **client's intellectual capability,** especially if written instructions are to be given. Next, take into account the client's **lifestyle** in order to incorporate his or her working hours, habits, diets, and support people into your teaching plan. **Knowing your own strengths, weaknesses,** and **knowledge level** provides an honest and comfortable approach to the teaching plan.

Knowledge deficit is a **nursing diagnosis** accepted by the North American Nursing Diagnoses Association and is applicable to the client in need of information.

After establishing the nursing diagnosis, the next step in the development of a teaching plan is setting goals. **Client goals** should specify time guidelines; should be realistic according to the client's cognitive, affective, and psychomotor abilities; and need not encompass everything there is to learn about the client's illness.

Nurses need to be familiar with **several teaching strategies** in order to meet the needs of individual clients. Lecture, demonstration and redemonstration, discussion, role modeling (demonstrating a certain attitude), pictures and models, pamphlets, learning games, audiovisual aids (videotapes, slides, films), puppetry, nursing textbooks, and the mass media (television, radio, newspapers) are teaching strategies nurses use for client teaching. Nurses employed as patient educators are available in many health-care agencies to assist with specific client teaching.

It is important to **educate the client's support people** also, such as parents of small children, spouses, or significant others.

Behavior modification is a teaching strategy using positive reinforcement or rewards for good behavior. Rewards may be praise, stars on a chart, or privileges.

DRILL AND PRACTICE QUESTIONS FOR REVIEW

Complete the statements below.

1. When a nurse is teaching a client the importance of deep breathing and coughing while the nurse is bathing the client, it is an example of _____ teaching.

2. When a nurse is teaching a seventh-grade class the dangers of alcohol and drug use, it is an example of _____, _____ teaching.

3. An early step in the client teaching process is establishing a harmonious relationship which is also called developing a _____ with the client.

4. When a nurse has determined the specific aspects of the topic to be learned by the client, the nurse has defined teaching _____.

5. Using gestures and facial expressions while teaching clients is called _____.

6. The final step of a teaching plan is _____.

7. Learning how to ride a bicycle is a _____ type of learning.

8. Learning how to calculate medication dosages is a _____ type of learning.

9. _____ learning would include changing a child's attitude about liking himself with a bald head after chemotherapy for cancer.

10. Using positive reinforcement in order to motivate learning is called _____.

Determine whether the following statements are TRUE or FALSE.

1. Lecture is an appropriate teaching strategy for the preschooler.

2. Persons who are ill often have short attention spans.

3. The nurse can use the same teaching strategy with various age groups as long as the subject is the same.

4. Teaching a client how to give a self-injection is best done on an informal basis.

5. Teaching a client how to perform a new skill two or three different ways is confusing.

6. School-age children have little difficulty learning abstract concepts.

7. It is important for a nurse to have a good knowledge base of the topics he or she is teaching.

8. Client learning goals should include time guidelines.

9. Drawing pictures is a useful visual aid when teaching children.

10. Group teaching is expensive, superficial, and often boring.

Determine the Type of Learning.

Determine the type of learning (affective, cognitive, psychomotor) in each of the situations below.

1. Mr. Razzano is learning how to read food labels for sodium content.

2. Mrs. Lee is learning to bathe her newborn.

3. Daniel, age three, is learning toilet training.

4. Mrs. Greenbaum is learning not to take responsibility for her husband's alcoholism.

5. Mrs. West is learning the list of precautions she must take because she is on anticoagulant therapy.

6. Mrs. Petri is learning how properly to apply her anti-emboli stockings.

7. Nathan, age four, is learning how to brush his teeth.

8. Nathan, age four, is learning to share is toys with playmates.

9. Jennifer, age sixteen, is learning which foods aggravate an acne condition.

10. Mr. Hansen is learning the medication schedule he should follow at home.

ANSWERS TO DRILL AND PRACTICE QUESTIONS

Completion Exercises

1. informal
2. formal, group
3. rapport
4. goals
5. nonverbal teaching
6. evaluation
7. psychomotor
8. cognitive
9. Affective
10. behavior modification

True/False Exercises

1. F
2. T
3. F
4. F
5. F
6. F
7. T
8. T
9. T
10. F

Identify the type of learning.

1. cognitive
2. psychomotor
3. psychomotor
4. affective
5. cognitive
6. psychomotor
7. psychomotor
8. affective
9. cognitive
10. cognitive

Chapter 28

COMPUTER USE IN NURSING

MAJOR NURSING CONCEPTS

A **computer system** includes many devices that work together in a synchronized fashion to process and store information. The three main categories of computer systems include **mainframes, minicomputers,** and **microcomputers.** A computer system commonly includes a **central processing unit** (processes information), **memory** (storage areas for information, which include disk and/or tape drives), and **peripherals** such as an **input device** (used to enter information into the computer system, e.g., a keyboard), and an **output device** (used to transfer information from the computer to the user, e.g., a monitor and/or printer). With the use of a **modem,** computers can "talk" to each other over phone lines. The equipment that comprises a computer system is referred to as computer **hardware.**

Computer **software** refers to special instructions, or programs written for, and executed by, a computer system. Commonly used computer software include **word processors** (for writing and editing of documents), **spreadsheets** (for business applications, grade computation), **data bases** (to store and sort information), **desktop publishing software** (sophisticated word processor), and **graphics software** (which creates pictures).

Computer systems are increasingly being used in health care for medical imaging (CT scans) and to facilitate and expedite laboratory analysis of specimens and the interpretation of diagnostic tests (such as ECG's). Sophisticated monitoring systems in intensive care settings utilize computer technology to determine physiologic parameters, display readings, monitor for abnormalities, and alert health care providers when life-threatening abnormalities occur. Generally, the above applications are **dedicated systems,** that is, the computer technology inherent in the system is not used for other applications.

Many hospitals use computer technology to facilitate the operation of the hospital and maintenance of patients' records. When computer terminals are networked to a central computer for this purpose the system is called a **hospital information system** (HIS). An HIS often includes a **nursing information system** that facilitates nursing assessment, documentation, and care planning. Information maintained on a computer is more legible and accessible than that in written records. With some systems, standardized nursing-care plans can be generated from the computer and individualized as appropriate. The confidentiality of patients' records must be ensured when computer systems for storage of patient information are developed. Nurses should be actively involved when plans are developed for an HIS.

With the use of **computer-assisted-instruction**(CAI) software, the education of students and health care consumers has been enhanced. CAI software includes **tutorials** (instructs the user in a content area), **drill and practice programs** (provide for repetitive testing of content already learned), and **simulations** (allow for application of previously learned knowledge in simulated situations). Computer programs are also used to facilitate **health risk appraisal** of consumers so that risks can be identified and suggestions for decreasing risk of major health problems be made.

121

With the use of computer systems and specialized software applications, administrative tasks, professional publishing, data base searching (to identify literature in a specific subject area), networking (collaboration with other professionals), and analysis of research data can also be accomplished.

DRILL AND PRACTICE QUESTIONS FOR REVIEW

Complete the statements below.

1. The equipment that comprises a computer system is called computer _____. Special instructions written for and executed by computer systems are called computer _____.

2. Mainframe computers are usually accessed through use of a computer terminal, which includes a _____ and a _____.

3. Personal computers belong to the category of computers known as _____.

4. To communicate with another professional by computer via telephone lines, a peripheral known as a _____ is necessary.

5. With the use of _____ software, a person can write and edit documents.

6. A computer system that is used for only one purpose is called a _____ system.

7. A network of computer terminals linked to a central computer to facilitate the operation of a hospital and the maintenance of patients' records is called a _____.

8. A hospital information system that includes a means for nursing assessment, planning, and documentation, incorporates a _____.

9. Computer-assisted instructional materials are categorized as _____, _____, _____, and _____.

10. A CAI program that permits users to test their ability to apply knowledge in mock situations is called a _____.

Determine whether the following statements are TRUE or FALSE.

1. With the computerization of patient records, the privacy of records cannot be insured.

2. Because of nurses' lack of expertise in computer technology, it is inappropriate that they be involved in the development of hospital information systems.

3. A nurse is preparing an article for publication in a nursing journal. A spreadsheet will facilitate the writing of the article.

4. The central processing unit of a computer system is primarily responsible for the processing and storage of information.

5. Many microcomputers have capabilities similar to larger computers.

6. A computer user enters information into a computer through the use of a specific device, such as a keyboard. Input devices, such as a keyboard, are also called peripherals.

7. A list of patients that are routinely seen by a nurse practitioner could be stored and sorted on a computer system with the use of data base software.

8. With the increasing use of computer systems for patient monitoring, the need for contact with human personnel will diminish.

9. The storage of patient records in a computer system is more efficient than storage in written charts.

10. Although people enjoy using CAI, its effectiveness as a teaching strategy has not been proven.

Identify each of the following as an example of computer hardware or computer software.

1. keyboard

2. monochrome monitor

3. modem

4. CRT

5. data base

6. mouse

7. CPU

8. disk drive

9. spreadsheet

10. graphics

ANSWERS TO DRILL AND PRACTICE QUESTIONS

Completion Exercises

1. hardware; software as programs

2. keyboard, display device (e.g., monitor)

3. microcomputer

4. modem

5. word processing

6. dedicated

7. hospital information system

8. nursing information system

9. games, tutorials, drill and practice programs, simulations

10. simulation

True/False Exercises

1.	F	6.	T
2.	F	7.	T
3.	F	8.	F
4.	T	9.	T
5.	T	10.	F

Identify Hardware/Software

1. hardware
2. hardware
3. hardware
4. hardware
5. software

6. hardware
7. hardware
8. hardware
9. software
10. software

PART VII

ASSESSMENT IN NURSING PRACTICE

Chapter 29

HEALTH ASSESSMENT: INTERVIEWING

MAJOR NURSING CONCEPTS

A **comprehensive health assessment** consists of three sections: health interview, physical assessment, and evaluation of diagnostic and laboratory data. The **interview** provides the focus and direction for the physical assessment, nursing diagnosis, nursing care plan, and implementation of care.

A **comprehensive health history** is lengthy and takes time to obtain. It includes the introduction, chief concern, history of present illness, past medical history, family medical history, and review of systems. If the client is a youngster, the comprehensive health history should also include any information concerning the pregnancy, birth, and neonatal history. Standardized agency nursing-history forms limit the information clients may offer.

It is important to have the **Introduction** before beginning the health history. The interviewer should introduce himself or herself, explaining the purpose of the interview and ascertaining whether the client is a child. It is also important to find out the name and relationship of the person to whom the interviewer will be talking.

The **Chief Concern (CC)** may be defined as the primary difficulty or problem that has brought the individual to the health-care agency. The chief concern is documented as a brief statement, using the client's own words in quotation marks. This statement may alert the nurse to any immediate nursing care that may be required (a client who states he feels warm may need his temperature taken).

The **History of Present Illness (PHI)** is a descriptive account of the chief concern. In order to identify and describe the problem more fully, the interviewer needs to know how long the problem has existed **(duration)**; the strength of the person's discomfort **(Intensity)**; how often the symptoms occur **frequency)**; what are the sequence, location, color, and odor of the symptoms **description)**; what are the symptoms that occur at the same time as the chief concern **(associated symptoms)**; what the client was doing at the onset of the initial symptoms; and what did the client do to try and alleviate the symptoms **person's actions)**.

The nurse is also concerned with the kind, amount, and frequency of medications taken to alleviate the chief concern or associated symptoms. At this time it is not wise to correct clients when you discover they are doing something wrong. Incorporating corrective actions into a teaching plan, to be shared at a later date, will help clients understand the problem and take corrective actions.

The **Client/Family Profile (PP or FP)** provides important psychosocial, financial, and personal data. It includes **identifying data** (name, birth date, age, religion, ability to pay bills,); **family pattern and structure** (how many people in family? how many lived at home? how many depend on client for support? life style); **living arrangements** (does client live in an apartment? single home? upstairs? downstairs? are living arrangements close to stores? transportation?); **occupational history** (past and current occupation); **educational history** (highest level of schooling); **cultural and religious heritage** (diet, expectations of health care and therapy); **economic status** (how will illness affect financial status?).

The **Past Medical History (PMH)** includes information about past illnesses that may influence the current level of health. Areas of concern include **childhood illnesses** (mumps, measles, chicken pox, rheumatic fever); **immunizations** (rubella—German measles— for women of childbearing age); **allergies** (sensitivities to foods and drugs, respiratory irritants); **illness** (if serious illness has occurred, ask for dates, treatments, complications); **accidents and injuries** (poisoning, falls, auto accidents); **health habits** (smoking, chewing tobacco, alcohol consumption, over-the-counter and prescription medications, sedentary or active lifestyle, last routine health examination, chest x-ray or dental exam); **prenatal history** for client under eighteen years of age.

The **Family Health History (FHH)** includes information on inherited diseases in the family. Health of siblings, children, parents, and grandparents are vital for a comprehensive health assessment.

The **Day History** includes information on nutrition, elimination, sleep patterns, recreation, interpersonal interactions, and sexual activity.

The **Review of Systems (ROS),** which is part of the health history, provides an overall assessment of the client to insure that all pertinent information has been elicited and documented. It should remain distinct and separate from the physical assessment.

The health history concludes with asking clients if they have any questions and setting up appointments for subsequent visits. Areas that need to be updated on follow-up visits include the introduction; identifying data (address, marital status); chief concern; history of present illness (duration, frequency, intensity, description, associated symptoms, and client action); interval history (events that have occurred since client was last seen); day history (update nutrition, elimination, developmental level, and life style information); conclusion (any problems the client wishes to discuss or seems concerned about).

After a thorough health-history interview, the nursing diagnosis is developed, followed by a nursing-care plan. Evaluation is continuous and may include obtaining further information on subsequent visits.

DRILL AND PRACTICE QUESTIONS FOR REVIEW

Completion Exercises

1. A comprehensive health assessment includes a _____, _____, and _____.

2. A comprehensive health history data base includes _____, _____, _____, _____, and _____.

3. A difficulty or problem that brings a client to the health-care agency is referred to as the _____.

4. Six areas of concern under the category of History of Present Illness are _____, _____, _____, _____, _____, and _____.

5. _____ symptoms are symptoms that occur at the same time as the chief concern.

6. The Family Health History is important because it lists any _____ in the family.

7. Information about a client's nutrition, elimination, sleep, and recreation patterns are part of the _____ History.

8. A final head-to-toe assessment is referred to as a _____.

True/False Exercises

1. Clients should never be asked to fill out a questionnaire as part of their health history interview.

2. Since note writing is distracting, nursing students should audiotape an interview with a client for the purpose of obtaining a health history.

3. The health history interview should begin with the chief concern.

4. During the interview, the nurse should form an opinion as to the client's reliability in order to offer an accurate health history.

5. The chief concern is the nurse's perception of what the client has told her or him.

6. Description of a chief concern includes the appearance of symptoms, its sequence, location, color, and odor.

7. What a client has done to try to alleviate symptoms is unimportant since the client will receive new medications for the symptoms.

8. Past illnesses influence the present level of health.

9. Medications can either cause or mask symptoms.

ANSWERS TO DRILL AND PRACTICE QUESTIONS

Completion Exercises

1. health interview, physical assessment, and evaluation of diagnostic and laboratory data

2. introduction, chief concern, history of present illness, past medical history, family medical history, and review of systems

3. chief concern

4. duration, intensity, frequency, description, associated symptoms, and person's actions

5. associated

6. inherited diseases

7. Day

8. review of systems

True/False Exercises

1. F
2. F
3. F
4. T

5. F
6. T
7. F
8. T
9. T

Chapter 30

HEALTH ASSESSMENT: PHYSICAL EXAMINATION

NOTE TO STUDENT

Be sure to review the illustrations and tables in this chapter. The figures provide graphic examples of specific assessment techniques and normal/abnormal findings. The tables summarize some of the most frequently utilized physical assessment skills.

MAJOR NURSING CONCEPTS

Findings obtained through **physical examination** (comprehensive examination or a selective examination) provide data that are utilized by nurses for the identification of client problems and nursing diagnoses.

The four techniques of physical examination include **inspection** (visual examination), **palpation** (touching), **percussion** (determination of the density of a body structure by striking a part with an examining finger), and **auscultation** (listening). Depending on the specific body part being examined and the assessment technique being utilized, specific equipment may be necessary (e.g., gloves when contact with body fluids is anticipated, stethoscope for auscultation, ophthalmoscope-otoscope for examining the eyes and ears). Principles of **comfort, safety, privacy,** and **asepsis** should be maintained throughout the physical examination.

Techniques of physical examination and findings **vary with age.** Children are particularly fearful of examination and equipment. Parental support and participation should be encouraged. Beginning with schoolage clients, a complete explanation of assessments to be performed is useful in alleviating anxiety. In conducting a physical examination, be alert to opportunities for teaching clients about self-breast or self-testicular examination.

A **comprehensive physical examination** generally begins with an inspection for general appearance (general impression of illness or wellness), a mental status assessment (orientation, mood, memory, anxiety level), and measurement of height, weight, and vital signs. Head circumference is measured until one year of age; chest and/or abdominal circumferences are measured only under special circumstances. The examination then generally proceeds from head to toe (except with infants and small children, when intrusive procedures are carried out first). Skin assessment is integrated throughout the complete physical exam and includes assessment of color, texture, turgor, and lesions.

DRILL AND DPRACTICE QUESTIONS FOR REVIEW

Complete the statements below.

1. The nurse auscultates for heart sounds at the left ventricle by placing the _____ of the stethoscope at the _____.

2. The Babinski reflex is elicited by _____. _____ would be considered an abnormal response.

3. A nurse suspects that a client has urinary retention. It would be appropriate to _____ the bladder for distention and _____ the bladder for a hollow sound.

4. Normal breath sounds include _____, _____, _____, and _____. Abnormal breath sounds include _____, _____, and _____. Breath sounds are best auscultated using the _____ of the stethoscope.

5. A nurse assesses a client's deep tendon reflexes and finds them to be hyperactive. They would be graded and recorded as _____.

6. The piece of equipment necessary to perform auscultation is the _____. High-pitched sounds are best heart with the _____, and low-pitched sounds are best heard with the _____.

7. A/an _____ temperature should be taken in a newborn infant. Heart rate should be determined at the _____ area.

8. When performing a comprehensive physical exam, a rectal exam should be performed in all persons over _____ years of age; women should have a pap smear every _____ years.

9. A child's height and weight are found to fall in the second percentile on a standardized growth chart. This finding should be reported to the physician because the child has the syndrome known as _____.

10. Measurement of chest circumference is made at the _____; measurement of abdominal circumference is made at the _____.

11. It is especially important to examine the hair of school-age children for _____, as evidenced by _____; it is especially important to examine the spine and back of preadolescents and adolescents for _____, as evidenced by _____.

12. A client has conjunctivitis. The conjunctiva would appear _____.

13. Visual-acuity testing is accomplished in persons who can identify the letters of the alphabet with the use of a _____ chart. The chart should be read at a distance of _____ feet. Normal vision for an adult is _____; for a preschool child _____.

14. In examination of the ear, the tympanic membrane normally appears _____ in color, and a _____ reflex is present.

15. Pain with flexion of the neck may be an indication of _____.

Determine whether the following statements are TRUE or FALSE.

1. A person complains of fever, barky cough, and sore throat. It is imperative that a tongue blade be used to examine the throat so that full visualization of the tonsils can be accomplished.

2. To alleviate anxiety during a physical exam, clients should be informed as to what you will be doing, and what they might feel before each assessment technique is initiated.

3. Dressings, bandaids, and another skin coverings should be left intact when skin assessment is performed.

4. Women should be taught to examine their breasts monthly immediately prior to their menstrual period.

5. To facilitate pelvic examination of a female client, a client should retain urine in a full bladder so that palpation of the ovaries can be accomplished.

State the techniques for examination of the following. Describe normal/abnormal findings.

1. skin turgor _____

2. PERL _____

3. Rinne test _____

4. fontanelles _____

5. bowel sounds _____

Situations

Situation 1

You are a pediatric nurse practitioner in private practice. Today you will be performing a comprehensive physical examination on two-year-old Jamie. State the order in which assessments will be performed. Describe how you will alleviate Jamie's anxiety about the examination.

Situation 2

Thirty-year-old Pat Jonson must be weighed daily. State the principles to be observed in obtaining her daily weight. Today she weighs 154 pounds. Her weight must be recorded in kilograms.

Situation 3

You are a nurse working on a medical unit where 23-year-old Jackie is recovering from viral pneumonia. Describe in detail the techniques you would utilize in carrying out a complete respiratory assessment.

ANSWERS TO DRILL AND PRACTICE QUESTIONS

Completion Exercises

1. diaphragm and then the bell, 4th or 5th intercostal space at the midclavicular line

2. striking the sole from the heel to the ball of the foot, flaring of the toes

3. palpate, percuss

4. vesicular, bronchovesicular, bronchial, rhonchi; rales, wheezing, stridor; diaphragm

5. 4+

6. stethoscope, diaphragm, bell

7. axillary; apical

8. 40; 3

9. failure to thrive

10. nipple line; umbilicus

11. pediculosis, yellow-white particles attached to hair strands and evidence of scratching the scalp; scoliosis, curvature of the spine in a standing or stooped-over position

12. reddened

13. Snellen; 20; 20/20; 20/50

14. pearly-grey; light

15. meningeal irritation

True/False Exercises

1. F
2. T
3. F
4. F
5. F

State the Technique

1. Lift a ridge of skin and observe if it falls back into place or not (with normal skin turgor, the skin returns to its prior position—with poor skin turgor, the skin remains in the lifted position).

2. Approach the uncovered eye from the side with a light and observe for pupillary constriction (normal).

3. After striking a tuning fork, hold the stem against the mastoid bone; after the sound is no longer heard, place the tuning fork in front of the ear canal; if the test is positive (normal), the sound will be heard again.

4. Palpate the skull for the anterior fontanelle (where the occipital, frontal, and parietal bones fuse) and the posterior fontanelle (where the occipital and perietal bones fuse). Normal fontanelles are neither tense nor depressed. The anterior fontanelle is normally present up to twelve to eighteen months of age; the posterior fontanelle closes at about two months of age.

5. Auscultate all four quadrants of the abdomen for a full minute to determine the presence of "pinging" sounds that normally occur every five to ten seconds.

Situations

Situation 1

To alleviate Jamie's anxiety:

- take time prior to the examination to become acquainted with him
- allow Jamie to handle some of the examining equipment
- encourage Jamie's parent to offer support during the examination
- talk to Jamie and keep him informed about what you are doing during the examination
- praise Jamie for cooperating during the examination

Order for the examination:

- general appearance
- mental status
- height, weight, vital signs (temperature, pulse, respiration; BP is **not** done on children before three years of age)
- examine the heart and lungs first, since crying, if it occurs later during the examination, can make it difficult to auscultate sounds
- head to toe assessment
- examination of the genitalia, ears, and throat should be done last, since these may precipitate fear and crying

Situation 2

Pat Jonson should be weighed on the same standing scale each day. Her weight should be taken at the same time each day (preferably before breakfast), and she should be wearing the same clothing (no shoes). Her weight of 154 pounds can be converted to kilograms by dividing 154 by 2.2 (1 kilogram = 2.2 lbs.). 154 pounds = 70 kilograms.

Situation 3

Respiratory assessment:

- count respirations for one full minute, noting ease or difficulty with respiration and whether or not accessory muscles are utilized
- percuss over lung tissue for normal resonant sounds, abnormal hyperresonant sounds (overinflated), or dull sounds (fluid-filled lung tissue)
- determine the diaphragmatic excursion by percussing the location of the bottom of the lungs as Jackie holds his breath, then percussing for the bottom of the lungs after Jackie exhales fully; the difference in these points is the diaphragmatic excursion
- auscultate breath sounds of each lobe, anteriorly and posteriorly; determine the presence/absence of sounds and whether sounds are normal or abnormal

Chapter 31

VITAL SIGNS

NOTE TO STUDENT

Procedures for obtaining temperature, pulse, respiration, and blood pressure are described throughout the chapter. Table 31-5 lists sites for arterial pulse taking; Table 31-6 describes factors that influence pulse rate; Table 31-7 lists abnormal pulse findings; and Table 31-10 lists factors that influence blood pressure.

MAJOR NURSING CONCEPTS

Vital signs (temperature, pulse, respiration, and blood pressure) are body process measurements needed to maintain life. An elevated or decreased body temperature reflects a disease process, with many implications for nursing. The narrow range for normal body temperature is 37 degrees to 38 degrees C or 96.8 degrees to 100.4 degrees F. This narrow range is maintained because of the balance between heat produced by the body and heat lost to the environment. **Heat** is produced and regulated by body metabolism. Body metabolism may be increased by muscular activity (exercise), fever, and increased oxidation of food. **Shivering** is muscular activity that raises body temperature. Methods of **heat loss** include conduction, convention, radiation and evaporation.

The internal or core temperature of the body, located in the thoracic and abdominal cavities, is referred to as **body temperature.** The **skin** has a lower temperature than the core temperature. **Hyperthermia** refers to elevated body temperature; **hypothermia** refers to lowered body temperature.

Factors that influence body temperature include the following:

- Age (newborns cannot shiver, and they have difficulty maintaining body temperature).

- External temperature (surrounding external air may affect internal temperature if the difference between the two is great).

- Circadian rhythm (body temperature is at its lowest between midnight and 6 a.m.; highest is between 4 and 8 p.m.).

- Exercise (increases metabolic rate).

- Hormone secretion (increased levels of thyroxine and growth hormone increase body metabolism).

- Psychological influence (stress increases the secretion of epinephrine and norepinephrine, which increase the metabolic rate).

- Hypothalmic regulation (the hypothalmus, considered the body's thermostat, initiates the stimulation for heat loss or heat production through vasoconstriction or shivering; the anterior section of the hypothalmus protects against hyperthermia, and the posterior portion protects against hypothermia).

- Neurological regulation (conscious awareness of the sensations of warmth or cold).

A **thermometer** (glass or electronic) measures body temperature. Glass thermometers register slowly, break easily (releasing mercury, which is (poison) and must be discarded after use or disinfected between patients. Electronic thermometers register quickly, do not contain mercury or glass, and eliminate the need for disinfection because of disposable covers.

Planning for temperature taking includes determining the best site (oral, rectal, or axillary) based on the age and condition of the client. **Axillary temperatures** are indicated for infants (rectal temperatures may cause damage to rectal mucosa), and recommended for toddlers and preschoolers because readings are accurate and less stressful. School-age children and adolescents may have oral temperatures. **Oral temperatures** should be taken only if the client is awake, alert, and cooperative. Contraindications to taking oral temperatures include confusion, children under five years of age, jaw surgery, mouth injury, mouth breathers, and people with mouth infections. Wait five minutes before taking oral temperatures when people have been smoking or drinking hot or cold beverages.

Glass rectal thermometers are inserted only the length of the glass bulb in infants, 1 inch in children, and 2 to 3 inches in adults. Similar insertion lengths apply to electronic thermometers. **Rectal temperature-taking** is contraindicated in newborns and for patients who have had rectal surgery or heart attacks.

The normal **axillary temperature** is 36.4 degrees C (97.6 degrees F). When a short-tipped glass thermometer is used, it requires approximately ten minutes to register.

Chemical thermometers (accuracy not well-documented) are temperature-recording strips that may be placed against the forehead or used as oral thermometers. They are disposable, register quickly, and are noninvasive.

Hypothermia or hyperthermia blankets permit continuous temperature monitoring by rectal-thermic probe or thermic leads taped onto the abdomen.

Pulse rate is an indirect measurement of the number of times the heart beats per minute. The heartbeat can usually be palpated and observed over the left fifth intercostal chest space, also known as the point of maximum impulse (PMI). The arterial pulse can usually be observed over the carotid artery (between trachea and sternocleidomastoid muscle), and the venous pulse can be observed over the jugular vein (lateral to the sternal notch). When assessing the heart rate and pulse, note rhythm, quality, and rate. Fetal heart sounds may be heard through the abdominal wall by using a doppler (ultrasonic instrument).

Pulse sites include the following:

- **Apical pulse:** Synonymous with heart rate. In fetuses and newborns, the rate may be up to 160 beats per minute; in adults the rate is usually up to 80 beats per minute. Apical pulse rate is indicated when client is receiving cardiac medicine or when peripheral pulse points are very weak.
- **Radial artery:** located at the inner surface of the wrist, it is the most common site used.
- **Brachial artery:** located in the inner surface of the elbow (antecubital fossa), it used is used to determine proper placement for stethoscope when taking blood pressure readings.

- **Temporal artery:** located in the area between the eye and the hairline, it is used when bruises or dressings obstruct radial site.
- **Carotid artery:** located lateral to the trachea at the level of the larnyx, it is used during cardiopulmonary resuscitation. Not routinely used for pulse measurements because external pressure (fingertips) may be interpreted by carotid artery receptors as increased blood pressure and in turn slow down the heart rate.
- **Femoral artery:** located on the medial side of the thigh.
- **Popliteal artery:** located in the popliteal fossa (back of the knee along the outer surface); not a common site for pulse assessment because it is sometimes difficult to locate.
- **Dorsalis pedis:** located on the top surface of the foot lateral to the extensor tendon of the large toe, it is used to determine circulation to the distal extremities.
- **Posterior tibial:** located behind the medial malleolus, it is used to assess circulation to lower extremities.

Abnormal heart and pulse rates include tachycardia (over 100 beats per minute) and bradycardia (less than 60 beats per minute).

Abnormal heart rhythms (arrhythmia) can be detected by listening to the apical heart rhythm or by pulse palpation. Sinus arrhythmia, found in children and adults, is a normal variation of rhythm that occurs when pressure changes in the chest during respiration. Premature beats (extra heart beats) may occur with emotional stress or in early pregnancy.

Quality of the heart rate refers to the strength or force of the contractions of the heart and to the presence of murmurs. Pulse quality may be recorded as 4+ (abnormally strong and bounding), 3+ (strong but not abnormal), 2+ (normal), or 0 (absent). **Pulse deficit,** which is the difference between the apical pulse rate and the radial pulse rate, may indicate weak or irregular ventricular contractions.

Respiratory rate refers to the number of inhalations and expirations a person takes in one minute. **Tachypnea** (respiratory rate above the average) can occur because of a lack of oxygen, while **bradypnea** (respiratory rate below the average) may occur when there is trauma to the respiratory center. **Dyspnea** is defined as difficult respirations, while **apnea** means cessation of respirations. **Respiratory assessment** includes rate, depth, rhythm, and evaluation of breath sounds. Normal breathing should be quiet and effortless.

Blood pressure is the force exerted by arterial blood against vessel walls. Changes in the heart rate, blood volume, or blood vessel resistance affect blood pressure. Receptors in the aortic arch and carotid artery are sensitive to blood pressure and will adjust by changing heart rate. **Hypertension** in adults exist when there is a persistent diastolic pressure over 90 mm Hg; **hypotension** in adults exists when the blood pressure is under 95/60. Factors that influence blood pressure include age, exercise, fever, exposure to cold, psychological stress, fluid overload, obesity, exposure to warmth, hemorrhage, anemia, and increased heart action. Blood pressure is measured indirectly by a **sphygmomanometer.** This measurement can be affected by exercise, psychological stress, or body position. Lower extremity blood pressure readings may be indicated when surgical dressings or intravenous therapy obstruct upper extremity sites. Direct blood pressure can be measured by insertion of a catheter into an artery. This technique may be indicated for clients with severe burns, heart failure, renal disease, or following heart surgery.

Factors that may lead to elevated or difficult-to-assess blood pressure measurements are auscultatory gaps, paradoxical blood pressure, orthostatic hypotension, supine hypotension, hypertension, and hypotension.

136

DRILL AND PRACTICE QUESTIONS FOR REVIEW

Completion Exercises

1. Body heat is maintained by a balance between _____ and _____.

2. The body's metabolic rate may be increased by _____, _____, and _____.

3. Four methods by which the body can lose heat are _____, _____, _____, and _____.

4. Internal body temperature refers to the temperature in the _____, _____, and _____.

5. _____ is an elevated temperature caused by external heating of the body.

6. Body temperature is influenced by _____, _____, _____, and _____.

7. _____ body temperature is done before the client begins to exercise.

8. The three common sites for temperature taking are _____, _____, and _____.

9. _____ is the average normal oral temperature.

10. _____ is the average normal rectal temperature.

11. _____ occurs when the heart contracts and pumps blood into the aorta.

12. _____ rate directly reflects heart rate.

13. The _____ artery should be used as a pulse site when there are obstructions at the radial site.

14. The major artery supplying blood to the head is the _____.

15. When assessing pulse rate, note _____, _____, and _____.

16. Tachycardia may be caused by _____, _____, _____, or _____.

17. Bradycardia may be caused by _____, _____, _____, or _____.

18. _____ are electrodes implanted in the heart that can stimulate a change in heart rate.

19. Blood pressure may be influenced by _____, _____, _____, or _____.

20. The difference between the systolic and diastolic blood pressure reading is referred to as the _____.

21. _____ hypotension may occur when rising too quickly to a standing position.

22. Three factors that may influence heart rate are _____, _____, and _____.

True/False Exercises

1. Vital sign measurements consist of temperature, pulse pressure, respiration, and blood pressure.

2. Humans are considered homeothermic beings.

3. Shivering lowers body temperature.

4. Skin has a higher temperature than the body's core temperature.

5. Temperature at birth is slightly lower than normal.

6. Newborns and older adults require extra external warmth in order to prevent chilling.

7. The body's circadian rhythm patterns are the same for all human beings.

8. Basal metabolism and body temperature are at its lowest point at 8 p.m.

9. Pain from external heat occurs at 113 degrees F (45 degrees C).

10. Electronic thermometers are based on the principle that mercury expands when heated.

11. When taking vital signs in an infant, always take respirations first.

12. Oral temperatures, using a glass thermometer, may be taken in children under six years of age.

13. Palpating both carotid arteries at the same time may cause a slow heart rate.

14. Pulse deficit is the difference between the apical pulse rate and the radial pulse rate.

15. Blood pressure is the force exerted by venous blood against the vessel wall.

Match the definitions with the following terms:

1. _____ two pulse waves for each heart beat   a. intermittent fever
2. _____ rhythm regular, strength alternatives between strong and weak   b. apical
3. _____ pulse located to the left of the trachea   c. dicrotic
4. _____ pulse located at the fifth intercostal space at the left midclavicular line   d. onset
5. _____ period of time during which temperature remains high   e. carotid
6. _____ pulse located at the inner surface of the wrist   f. stadium
7. _____ irregularly regular beat   g. relapsing fever
8. _____ temperature alternates between elevated and normal levels on a day-to-day basis   h. pulse alterans
9. _____ temperature always elevated but high levels vary   i. radial
10. _____ gradual rise in temperature   j. bigeminal
11. _____ loss of body heat from a warmer to a cooler object by direct contact   k. remittent
12. _____ loss of body heat to moving air   l. temporal

13. _____ loss of body heat because of air conditioning

    m. conduction

14. _____ loss of body heat by profuse sweating

    n. evaporation

    o. radiation

    p. convection

Situations

Situation 1

Tom who is three months old, was admitted to the hospital because he has had a fever for five days. As the nurse caring for him, list the order in which you would take his vital signs, state the appropriate route for temperature-taking, and describe the procedure for temperature measurement.

Situation 2

Mrs. smith, age thirty-five, needs to have her pulse taken before the nurse can administer cardiac medication. Describe the procedure for obtaining a radial pulse, and include the rationale for each step.

Situation 3

John Winter is a seventy-year-old man hospitalized for hypertension. He weighs 200 pounds, ambulates slowly, and his blood pressure is 186/94. His pulse rate is 96. He tells you that he rarely exercises and that he has frequent severe headaches. His physician has left instructions to be notified if his blood pressure goes above 220/100 or below 130/80. Mr. Winter is on special medication to lower his blood pressure and medication to relieve his headaches. As the nurse caring for him, discuss how age, obesity, and exercise influence blood pressure; list three possible problems and solutions, that may occur when using blood pressure equipment; and develop an appropriate nursing care plan.

ANSWERS TO DRILL AND PRACTICE EXERCISES

Completion Exercises

1. heat produced by the body and then lost to the environment

2. muscular activity (exercise), fever, increased sympathetic nerve stimulation, increased secretions of thyroxine or increased oxidation of food

3. conduction, convection, radiation, and evaporation

4. thoracic and abdominal cavities and the central nervous system

5. hyperthermia

6. age, external temperature, circadian rhythm, exercise, hormone secretions, hypothalmic regulation, neurological regulation, or psychological influence

7. basal

8. oral, rectal, and axillary

9. 98.6 degrees F; 37.6 degrees C

10. 99.6 degrees F; 37.6 degrees C

11. systole

12. apical pulse

13. temporal

14. carotid

15. rate, rhythm, and quality

16. exercise, fever, hypoxemia, low blood pressure, stress, or pain

17. poor conduction through the heart, vagal nerve stimulation, bronchial suctioning, or forceful vomiting

18. cardiac pacemakers

19. age, exercise, fever, blood volume, obesity, heart action, or anemia

20. pulse pressure

21. orthostatic

22. age, sex, exercise, psychological state, body temperature, blood volume, and body position

True/False Exercises

1.	F	8.	F
2.	T	9.	T
3.	F	10.	F
4.	F	11.	T
5.	F	12.	F
6.	T	13.	T
7.	F	14.	T
		15.	F

Matching

1.	c	8.	a
2.	h	9.	k
3.	e	10.	d
4.	b	11.	m
5.	f	12.	p
6.	i	13.	o
7.	j	14.	n

Situations

Situation 1

- Respiration, pulse, blood pressure, and temperature
- Axillary, using either an electronic thermometer or glass thermometer

Procedure for taking axillary temperature:

- Use a short-tipped, glass thermometer or an electronic thermometer.
- Wash hands, identify patient, and explain procedure. This process prevents transmission of microorganisms, ensures the patient's safety, and elicits patient's cooperation.
- Place the bulb of the glass thermometer within the axillary and gently hold Tom's arm close to his body. For patient safety, do not leave the patient while thermometer is in place.
- Hold thermometer in place for approximately ten minutes. Electronic thermometers are highly recommended since they register in less than ten seconds and do not expose the patient to possible damage of broken glass.

Situation 2

This is the procedure for taking a radial pulse:

- Wash your hands, identify the patient, and explain procedure to the patient. This process prevents transmission of microorganisms and ensures the patient's safety and cooperation.
- Position the patient comfortably. When the patient is resting, an accurate reading may be obtained.
- Place three fingers lightly on inner aspect of wrist over radial artery. Never use your thumb, because it has its own pulse.
- Count the pulse for fifteen seconds and multiply by four. This will give you the beats per minute. If the pulse is irregular, count for one minute.
- Evaluate the pulse strength (full, bounding, weak, thready) and rhythm (regular, irregular). Irregularities may indicate cardiovascular problems.
- Record rate, strength, and rhythm. Documentation is necessary and required in order to communicate the patient's status to others.

Situation 3

Blood pressure is influenced by the following:

- **Age:** With increasing age, there is greater circulatory space, which results in more force necessary to move blood around. This increases blood pressure.
- **Obesity:** Since more force from the heart is needed to move blood through a larger system, blood pressure is increased.
- **Exercise:** This increases the stroke volume of the heart, thereby increasing blood pressure.

Three possible problems that may occur with blood pressure equipment:

- **Inaccurate reading:** This may be due to cuff size. The cuff should be no wider than two thirds of the upper arm width. A wider cuff may give a false low reading; a narrow cuff may give a false high reading.
- **Inaudible Korotkoff's sounds:** Test the stethoscope, and point ear pieces forward.
- **Cuff does not inflate:** Check tubings, connections and valve.

Nursing Care Plan:

Assessment:

- B/P 186/94. Respiratory rate 96. Patient ambulates slowly for short periods of time. Complains of severe, frequent headaches, and is overweight for his age and body frame.

Nursing Diagnosis:

- Alteration in comfort, and pain (headache) related to increased blood pressure.

Goal:

- Patient will obtain relief from headache.

Criteria:

- Patient verbalizes about a decrease in frequency and intensity of headaches.

Nursing orders:

1. Assess blood pressure at least q4h.

2. Take blood pressure before administering medication to lower blood pressure (antihypertensive medication)

3. Notify physician if blood pressure goes above 220/100 or below 130/80.

4. Teach patient how to rise slowly from a supine position in order to prevent a sudden drop in blood pressure.

5. Ask patient to inform you whenever he has a headache, and ask him to be specific about location and severity, on a scale of 0–5 (0 = no pain; 5 = worst pain).

6. Administer pain medication as ordered.

Chapter 32

LABORATORY ASSESSMENT

MAJOR NURSING CONCEPTS

Nurses can gather important information about their clients' health from **diagnostic-laboratory studies.** In addition to improving your nursing care, results from laboratory studies verify medical diagnoses and determine the effectiveness of treatment.

Preparation for diagnostic-laboratory procedures often include **physical measures** (enemas, NPO status, medications), informed **consent,** and a thorough **explanation** to the client in an effort to alleviate fears and anxieties.

Nursing diagnoses related to diagnostic procedures may include knowledge deficit related to the purpose or preparation for the procedure, anxiety, potential for injury, and alteration in comfort.

Painful and possibly harmful procedures are done only when absolutely necessary on the **infant.** To provide support the parents should accompany the baby, but they should not help with the procedure. Infants should be picked up and comforted when the procedure is finished. Because of their fear of pain, **toddlers** and **preschoolers** need only short explanations immediately before the procedure is scheduled.

The **school-ager** and **adolescent** cooperate more readily, especially if they are given clear explanations. Adolescents who seem mature and **adults** who appear "in control" may be frightened and also need reassurance. The **older adult** is easily exhausted by diagnostic procedures, especially when they are lying on hard examining tables or when their sclerotic veins make blood sampling difficult.

Nursing responsibility for diagnostic-laboratory study involves ascertaining that the physician has obtained informed consent; scheduling the procedure; explanation to client and support people; physical and psychological preparation; possibly transporting client to appropriate department; providing support during the procedure; evaluating the client's response to the procedure; documenting completion of the procedure; and perhaps aftercare of equipment and specimens.

Blood-drawing is the most common laboratory procedure done because analysis of blood produces a great deal of information about one's health status. Explain to the client that the procedure stings and that only a proportionately small amount of blood is being withdrawn. Gloves should be worn when drawing blood to protect oneself from exposure to AIDS and hepatitis.

The CBC (**complete blood count**) yields information about the major components of the blood. See Appendix G for normal values of the following components. The WBW (**white blood cell count**) supplies information about the immune system. The **differential** count examines the different kinds and numbers of white blood cells. The RBC (**red blood cell**) count is a gross determination of the number of red blood cells present, while the **hematocrit** determines the ratio of red blood cells to plasma volume. The **hemoglobin** reflects the oxygen-carrying ability of the red blood cells. **Reticulocytes** are immature red blood cells being produced, and their presence is usually a healthy sign.

The ESR **(erythrocyte sedimentation rate)** is the rate at which red blood cells settle in the plasma; an increased rate is indicative of an inflammation. **Hemoglobin S** is type of hemoglobin found in people with sickle cell anemia (red blood cells are concave in shape and therefore cannot carry oxygen in adequate amounts).

The client does not have to be NPO for a CBC, but the client must be NPO in the morning for blood chemistry studies.

Blood may be drawn from a vein **(venipuncture),** an artery **(arteriopuncture),** or **capillary** (finger, heel, earlobe). See Figure 32-2 for commonly used venipuncture sites, and Figure 32-1 for techniques of venipuncture. The radial artery. brachial artery, and the femoral artery are most often used for arteriopunctures. Arteriopunctures are usually done to analyze the blood's gases. Although applying pressure to the puncture site after needle withdrawal is important after a venipuncture (two to three minutes), applying pressure to an arteriopuncture site (ten minutes) is extremely important in order to prevent bleeding.

Studies involving electrical impulses include the **electrocardiogram,** which detects normal and abnormal electrical impulses from the heart, especially irregular heartbeats; and the **stress electrocardiography,** which is a cardiogram taken while the client exercises. Electrophysiology studies involve positioning a catheter in the heart in order to identify abnormal heartbeats (arrhythmias) and determine the best treatment. The **electroencephalogram** EEG record the electrical impulses of the brain. An **electromyogram** is a long and sometimes painful procedure which involves the insertion of small needles into the muscles and the electrical stimulation of the muscles in order to study muscular activity.

X-rays may be done with or without the use of **contrast media.** Contrast media is dye which can be injected into a vein, travels to a specified organ, and then the X-rays are taken. The radio-opaque contrast medias often cause the client to experience a hot flash, and some individuals may develop allergic reactions to these iodine-based dyes. See Table 32-2 for symptoms of a person with iodine sensitivity. It is important to protect yourself from over-exposure to radiation by leaving the room before the X-rays are taken or by wearing a lead apron if you absolutely must stay in the room. Some commonly performed X-ray procedures include **mammography** (radiographic study of breast tissue), **computerized tomography** (CT Scan), and **fluoroscopy** (several successive X-rays in the format of a moving picture).

Magnetic resonance imaging (MRI) uses no radiation and gives clear images of soft tissue (without contrast media), using magnetic fields and radio waves. Ultrasound (echograms) uses high frequency sound waves to record a pattern or image of body tissues.

Aspiration is an often painful technique for withdrawing body tissue or fluid using a specially designed needle. A **lumbar puncture** (spinal tap) is the most common aspiration procedure done and involves removing cerebral spinal fluid from the spinal canal for analysis. The client scheduled for a lumbar puncture needs supportive teaching regarding the safety of the procedure. During the procedure, strict sterile technique is adhered to; the client is helped to assume and maintain a vertabrae separating position (see Figures 32-15A and 32-15B); fluid is withdrawn for analysis; and occasionally pressure readings are obtained and medications are administered into the spinal canal. Advise the client to stay flat in bed for four to eight hours after the procedure to prevent spinal headaches. When bone marrow is removed for analysis, the procedure is called a **bone marrow aspiration.** Removal of fluid from the pleural cavity **thoracentesis)** and a **paracentesis** (removal of fluid from the peritoneal cavity) are also aspiration studies.

Biopsy is a diagnostic procedure involving the removal of a sample of body tissue for analysis. Bone, liver, and kidney (renal) are commonly biopsied sites.

Direct internal visualization of a body part is called **endoscopy** (gastroscopy studies the stomach, bonchoscopy studies the bronchi, etc.). These procedures are often frightening for the client, and the nurse needs to offer support, aid in body positioning, observe the client for untoward effects, and assess the client after the procedure for discomfort and signs of any damage caused by pressure from the instrumentation.

Nuclear medicine studies involve the ingestion or injection of a radioactive substance which will accumulate in a specific organ (the thyroid, for example) and allow visualization by scintillation (type of Geiger counter). Although the dose of radiation is small, these studies should not be used with pregnant women, and lactating mothers should stop breast feeding until the substance is completely excreted from the body. This client should not be cared for by pregnant health-care personnel for forty-eight hours after the procedure in order to protect the health care worker from exposure to radiation.

Nurses often are responsible for collecting body fluids to send to the laboratory to determine if microorganisms are present and which antibiotics are effective against the microorganisms. Gloves should be worn to protect yourself from contamination, and you must use sterile techniques to obtain the specimen so no further organisms are added to the specimen accidentally.

While someone else may have performed the actual diagnostic study, it is often the nurse's responsibility to document the client's response to the procedure, to describe the specimens obtained, and to assess for untoward effects such as bleeding, anxiety, fear, pain, or discomfort.

DRILL AND PRACTICE QUESTIONS FOR REVIEW

Complete the statements below.

1. The most important reason for encouraging a parent to accompany an infant during a diagnostic procedure is so that the parent can provide _____.

2. Recording an ECG during exercise is called a _____.

3. A common sensation experienced by clients after the injection of a radio-opaque dye is _____.

4. The differential count examines _____ blood cells.

5. Three sites commonly used for arteriopunctures are the _____, the _____, and the _____ arteries.

6. Following an arteriopuncture, the nurse should apply pressure to the puncture site for _____ minutes.

7. An _____ describes the electrical impulses in the brain.

8. Electromyograms study the electrical potential of _____.

9. If a dye is to be injected, the nurse should first determine if the client is allergic to a common untrient called _____.

10. Radiographic examination of the breast is called _____.

11. Successive X-rays similar to moving pictures are referred to as _____.

12. A noninvasive diagnostic procedure using soundwaves is called _____ or _____.

13. A _____ is an aspiration study of the cerebral spinal fluid.

14. During a lumbar puncture, the infant is positioned in a _____ position, and the adult in a _____ position.

15. Aspiration of fluid from the peritoneal cavity is called a _____.

16. _____ technique is used when obtaining a specimen for culture and sensitivity.

Determine whether the following statements are TRUE or FALSE.

1. It is the nurse's legal responsibility to answer a client's questions about the risks and benefits of diagnostic procedures.

2. The nurse can eliminate all fear by informing the client exactly what will happen during a diagnostic procedure.

3. Following any frightening or painful procedure, an infant should be picked up and cuddled.

4. In order to develop trust, detailed instructions are useful in preparing the toddler for a diagnostic procedure.

5. Most adolescents do not need reassurance before or during a diagnostic procedure because they have reached a significant level of maturity.

6. Providing for rest periods following diagnostic studies is an important part of a nursing care plan for older adult clients.

7. Repeated explanations of diagnostic procedures may be necessary because anxiety and stress may prevent the client from understanding everything at one time.

8. Clients having diagnostic procedures performed one day after the other may become dehydrated.

9. Clients preparing themselves at home for diagnostic procedures should have written instructions.

10. Children need not be accompanied to a strange department for a diagnostic procedure if their ID band is secure and clearly visible.

11. During a procedure, it is helpful to ask the client casual questions to divert his or her attention.

12. Arterial blood may be drawn from the heel or earlobe.

13. A client should be NPO for a CBC (complete blood count).

14. Pressure to the puncture site following a venipuncture is unnecessary.

15. Signs of allergic reaction to a radiographic contrast media include itching, hives, and difficulty of breathing.

16. Aspiration of fluid from the pleural cavity is referred to as a thoracentesis.

Situation

Mr. North is admitted to the hospital for a bronchoscopy. He is forty-eight years old and has had a recurrent and worsening cough for many months. This is Mr. North's first admission to a hospital. He tells the nurse, "Even though I have been smoking for twenty years, I never thought I would get sick." List several nursing interventions you would include in Mr. North's care plan specific to his impending bronchoscopy.

ANSWERS TO DRILL AND PRACTICE EXERCISES

Completion Exercises

1. support
2. stress electrocardiography
3. a hot flash
4. white
5. radial, brachial, femoral
6. ten
7. electroencephalogram
8. muscles
9. iodine
10. mammography
11. fluoroscopy
12. ultrasound or echogram
13. lumbar puncture
14. sitting, side-lying
15. paracentesis
16. Sterile

True/False Questions

1.	T	9.	T
2.	F	10.	F
3.	T	11.	F
4.	F	12.	F
5.	F	13.	F
6.	T	14.	F
7.	T	15.	F
8.	T	16.	T

Situation

In preparing Mr. North for a bronchoscopy, the following interventions should be included:

- ascertaining the informed consent was obtained;
- scheduling the procedure (may be done by a physician);
- explanation of procedure to Mr. North and his family;
- physical preparation (NPO, sedative) and psychological preparation (repeated explanations if necessary, allowing Mr. North to verbalize concerns);
- accompanying him to and supporting him during the procedure;
- continuous assessments during the procedure such as vital signs, anxiety levels, and skin color; and
- careful description of Mr. North's condition during and after the procedure (vital signs, especially respirations, skin color, pain, and additional fears)

PART VIII

PROMOTING HEALTH, GROWTH, AND WELL-BEING

Chapter 33

PROVIDING A POSITIVE, THERAPEUTIC ENVIRONMENT

MAJOR NURSING CONCEPTS

People respond to change in their environment and meet their basic needs because they are in constant interaction with both their internal environment (body) and their external environment (surroundings). This continuous interaction occurs by means of the individual's five senses (visual, auditory, tactile, olfactory, gustatory) and an intact, functioning central nervous system.

People orient themselves to their surroundings and sense whether they are upright or lying down; by proprioception (an ability to sense shape and distance of objects) and an intact, functioning vestibular mechanism in the inner ear.

The sense of **touch** enables people to determine the size, consistency, and texture of objects. **Auditory** receptors help us not only to hear sounds but to determine their distance. To help people respond to potentially dangerous situations very quickly (touching a hot saucepan), the **sensory stimulus** goes directly to the spinal cord and immediately evokes a motor response (removing hand quickly). This stimulus, however, continues on to the cerebral center, where it is interpreted and enables the person to realize she or he has been burned. People who do not have a functioning intact nervous system experience a confusing, frightening world.

Stimulus refers to an agent or factor that can be perceived by sensory receptors, while **stimulation** is the arousal or inciting to activity as a result of the stimulus. The stimulus may be physical (touching dry ice), psychological (passing state boards), social (marriage), or sensory (light from a camera flash). The **four categories of stimulation include** sensory, cognitive, social, and physical; the three levels of response are emotional, cognitive, and motor.

Sensory stimulation is needed constantly in order for the human being to develop and function competently. Individuals who have one or more senses that are weak or not functioning (sight) tend to strengthen another sense (hearing) to fill the need for stimulation. Impaired sensory stimulation may be the result of neurological problems, and careful assessment is required. Hearing is considered the last sense lost as individuals lapse into unconsciousness, and it is thought to be the first sense regained.

Cognitive stimulation (puzzles, riddles, problem-solving questions) create interest and excitement because they require the attention of the listener and the ability to think at different levels.

Social stimulation, which results from interactions with other individuals, goes beyond simple sensory or cognitive stimulation because it brings about a level of satisfaction or contentment that cannot be achieved in any other way. Nurses should be concerned about patients who do not receive visitors during their hospitalization or patients who have no relatives or friends to help them when they are ready for discharge. Loneliness or separation from others may inhibit social stimulation and social interaction.

Physical stimulation may be **environmental** (walking slowly on a hot day, learning to ice-skate), or it may be **protective** (moving quickly away from a running dog). **Physical stimulation** increases body activity and reduces stress.

Sensory deprivation refers to an environment lacking adequate sensory, social, physical, or cognitive stimulation. This type of environment causes people to lose their ability to orient themselves as to time and place and reduces their ability to think logically and appropriately.

Sensory overload occurs when individuals are surrounded by or receive more stimulation than can be tolerated or processed. This type of environment can occur in intensive-care units when bright lights are never turned down; when machines are constantly making loud noises; and when there are no windows so that one cannot determine whether it is day or night. In addition, sensory overload may occur when students have too many assignments that are all due within a short time. Individuals with **sensory overload act confused and fatigued, and may be unable to make rational decisions.**

The **assessment** of the individual for **stimulation needs** begins with sensory status:

- vision
- hearing
- touch
- taste
- smell

Physical age is then compared with chronological age. Assessment of equipment that may limit ambulation (cane, cast) or a medical diagnosis that may require prolonged periods of inactivity is also considered.

Low birth-weight infants, premature infants, children separated from their parents, children with a poor parent-child relationship, people on bed rest, and patients on isolation precautions for contagious diseases tend to suffer from sensory deprivation and need to have these needs assessed.

People on medication to reduce sensory input (sedatives) may be unaware of stimulating factors in their environment. They may need frequent orientation to time and day of the week as well as a reduction in visits from relatives, friends, or significant others.

Older adults with visual, auditory, or taste loss may suffer from sensory deprivation. This situation may be alleviated if they can join groups and become active in physical therapy and recreational type programs.

People with **distorted reality** (delusions—misinterpreting something that is actually there; hallucinations—seeing or hearing things that only they can see or hear) may need to have stimuli reduced so that they are exposed to fewer sights or sounds that can easily be misinterpreted.

Analysis continues with the formulation of appropriate nursing diagnoses and client goals. The nurse should be aware that stimulation deprivation or overload is easy to overlook when caring for patients with multiple serious physical problems.

A **nursing diagnosis** related to sensory status is:

- Sensory perceptual alteration.

Planning and implementation include writing specific nursing orders for increasing or reducing stimulation. Nurses sometimes believe that "only talking" to patients is not doing nursing. This time is very important to clients, since it may be their only interaction for the day.

The need for stimulation differs over the life span.

1. **Infants** experience the world around them by using their already-developed five senses. Newborns follow objects, respond to touch, and can distinguish between sweet and bitter tastes. Infants usually resist new tastes, respond intensely to touch, and require holding. At about three months of age infants learn to recognize the same people, and by four months of age they are unhappy when you leave them. Hospitalized infants require active motor stimulation and social, one-to-one stimulation.

2. **Toddlers and preschoolers** respond best to activities that require touch or manipulation. Books, colored pictures, and visual and auditory nursery rhymes can keep this age group occupied for long periods of time. Preschoolers reflect interest in their environment by asking many questions. Different size boxes and pegs suit their need for manipulation. Security needs are also very important to this age group. Toddlers and preschoolers discriminate in their interactions, and they make new friendships if parents are close by. **Cognitive stimulation** can be accomplished with picture puzzles, pencil-and-paper games, clay or play dough, and fingerpaints. **Social interaction** can be achieved by taking hospitalized preschoolers to other hospital units and engaging them in activities with other children.

3. The **school-ager and adolescent** need hearing stimulation as well as intellectual stimulation since they easily become bored. They enjoy short-term projects with a reward and a sense of accomplishment at the end. Ill children regress when they are ill, so certain competitive type activities may only frustrate the child rather than stimulate. Adolescents require interaction with other sin order to meet their social and cognitive stimulation needs. Activities for this group include active motion skill games and short homework assignments.

4. The **young and middle-aged adult** have already developed a comfortable sensory stimulation level. By this time they have become work-oriented, and many like to spend time on projects. Adults are interested in their community and the world around them. Hospitalized adults may be interested in watching television, reading newspapers, or reading books, while others may be interested in needlepoint or painting.

5. The **older adult** may become sensory-deprived because advancing age may cause less acute eyesight or fading taste sensation. The sensation of touch and cognitive and intellectual stimulation and functioning remains intact. The older adult's need for sleep may be the result of boredom or lack of stimulation rather than from physical need. Needlework, knitting, rug punching, chess, or checkers are cognitive and physical stimulation activities that offer a sense of achievement and improve self-esteem. Pets also offer a special kind of interaction for the older adult.

Reducing stimuli for the patient with sensory overload may include diminishing bright lights; reducing unnecessary verbal interaction between staff personnel; limiting visitors; and transferring the patient to a quieter room. The nurse should explain all procedures and repeat instructions and explanations as often as necessary. This process enables the patient to clarify the stimuli and keep a sense of personal control.

Evaluation includes looking at the patients' level of stimulation within their total environment of care.

DRILL AND PRACTICE QUESTIONS FOR REVIEW

Completion Exercises

1. The five senses that enable the average person to interact with his or her environment are _____, _____, _____, _____, and _____.

2. _____ in the inner ear and _____ help people to orient themselves in space.

3. The four types of stimulation may be categorized as _____, _____, _____, and _____.

4. Puzzles and problem-solving situations are two examples of _____ stimulation.

5. _____ stimulation comes from interactions with other people.

6. When the environment lacks sufficient stimuli to maintain sensory, social, physical, or cognitive stimulation, _____ _____ occurs.

7. _____ _____ occurs when a person receives more sensory stimulation than she or he can tolerate.

8. When assessing clients for stimulation needs, the first category to be assessed should be _____ status.

9. Infants separated from their parents may develop symptoms of _____ _____.

10. Failure-to-thrive children require _____ stimulation and a _____ _____ relationship.

11. _____ are disturbances in perception or a false belief.

True/False Exercises

1. Sensory stimuli always go directly to the cerebral cortex without passing through the spinal cord.

2. It is not necessary to have mental and physical stimulation every day, since individuals do not need it to develop and function adequately.

3. Sensory stimulation from the muscles or body organs is one of the protective ways the body is alerted to injury.

4. As people lapse into unconsciousness, the last sense lost is vision.

5. Sensory deprivation and overload cause similar changes in behavior.

6. People on bedrest are cognitively stimulated by many hours of television viewing.

7. People with hearing or visual deficits are not prone to sensory deprivation because other senses become stronger.

8. Establishing daily routines, reducing overhead lighting, and decreasing sounds are three ways to reduce sensory deprivation.

9. Hallucinations are things people see or hear that are unfounded or unreal in the environment.

10. Introducing new and different foods to the hospitalized client is an effective way to increase stimulation.

Situations

Situation 1

Mrs. Jackson, a seventy-five-year-old patient, had surgery one week ago to repair a fracture of her left leg. She is in a private room; her left leg is in a cast, and she finds it very difficult to move around in the bed. She is irritable, anxious, and disoriented as to day, time, and place. She states that she "has no appetite to eat." List an appropriate nursing diagnosis, and state at least four nursing actions that could be used to manage Mrs. Jackson's sensory alterations.

Situation 2

Mr. Gray, a fifty-year-old patient, is in the intensive care unit because he has had a heart attack. For the last four days he has exhibited signs of confusion as to day, time, and place; irritability with family and staff personnel; difficulty in sleeping and slowed ability to think through simple problems. List an appropriate nursing diagnosis, and state at least four nursing actions that could be used to manage Mr. Gray's sensory alterations.

ANSWERS TO DRILL AND PRACTICE EXERCISES

Completion Exercises

1. sight, hearing, touch, taste, and smell

2. vestibular mechanisms, proprioception

3. sensory, cognitive, social, and physical

4. cognitive

5. social

6. sensory deprivation

7. sensory overload

8. sensory

9. maternal deprivation

10. cognitive; warm, reassuring, caring

11. delusions

True/False Exercises

Situations

Situation 1

Nursing diagnosis: Actual sensory-perceptual alteration related to confining illness (sensory deprivation). Nursing interventions that may be used to alleviate sensory deprivation are as follows:

- provide a calendar and a clock to reorient patient to time, day, and place
- provide different types of growing plants
- provide some type of appropriate diversional therapy—needlepoint, knitting
- move client closer to activity, and avoid isolation of client
- encourage activity and exercise
- control discomfort or pain
- provide cognitive stimulating games—cards, if appropriate
- encourage loner visits by friends, family, and staff personnel
- offer reassurance by touching patient (if culture permits)
- use television or radio only to the point that it does not become monotonous
- explain all procedures
- provide continuity of care by the same personnel as often as possible

Situation 2

Nursing diagnosis: Actual sensory-perceptual alteration related to intensive care unit environment (sensory overload). Nursing actions that may be used to alleviate sensory overload include the following:

- provide dim lighting, if possible, especially at night; provide eye covering
- reduce conversations at the bedside—keep explanations of procedures and treatments short and simple
- provide soft music through earphones
- plan nursing care in order to provide for uninterrupted rest periods and sleep
- limit visitors and limit their length of stay
- control discomfort and pain
- teach relaxation exercise
- provide clock and calendar
- place patient near window, if possible

Chapter 34

COMFORT AND SAFETY

NOTE TO STUDENT

Be sure to review the tables on Environmental Hazards and Safety Precautions by Age Group.

MAJOR NURSING CONCEPTS

Comfort refers to freedom from pain and a sense of well-being. People react to discomfort differently, depending on their culture, sex role, and general background, as well as the trust they feel in those around them.

Therapeutic environments foster a sense of comfort and well-being. Adequate ventilation, comfortable temperature (68-74 degrees), appropriate humidity, freedom from noise, and appropriate light contribute to a therapeutic external environment. Providing for peoples' privacy, insuring the safety of their personal property, and allowing them some sense of control also contribute to maintenance of a sense of well-being.

Pain is a subjective feeling of distress in response to some form of tissue injury. It is a protective mechanism. The pain impulse originates at the site of tissue injury and is transmitted to the brain via the spinal cord. Pain perception occurs in the brain, and voluntary action in response to pain is also mediated by the brain. Pain impulses originating at peripheral nerves also elicit the **withdrawal** (involuntary) reflex.

According to the **gate control theory of pain,** sensory nerves that transmit pain impulses are composed of small fibers (stimulated by noxious, pain-producing stimuli) and large fibers (easily stimulated by stimuli such as massage and pressure). The stimulation of large fibers can prevent transmission of impulses from more noxious stimuli, thus preventing perception of pain. Many measures to alleviate pain are successful due to stimulation of large fibers.

Pain stimulates the **sympathetic nervous system,** activating the fight-or-flight response, which increases vital functions and mobilizes the body to deal with stress. Very severe pain precipitates nausea, vomiting, and fainting, as the body is unable to cope. Pain also activates the **endorphin system** (natural opiate-like substances), which helps alleviate pain.

Nursing **assessment** with regard to pain involves the determination of individual factors that might contribute to pain (anxiety and educational level, previous experiences with pain, feelings about using pain meds). When assessing a person in pain, it is important to determine the **duration, frequency, intensity,** and **full description** of the pain. Pain can be described as **acute** (intense, short-lived), **chronic** (lasting longer than six months), **intermittent, persistent, intractable** (uncontrollable), **referred** (originates in a part of the body other than where it is felt), or **phantom** (experienced in a part of the body that has been amputated).

Nursing diagnoses pertinent to the pain experience include the following:

- Alteration in comfort: pain
- Alteration in comfort: chronic pain

Planning and implementation strategies to prevent or alleviate pain include **cutanous stimulation, distraction,** measures to **reduce anxiety,** and general **comfort measures** (e.g., providing for clean, wrinkle-free linen). In addition, the administration of prescribed **analgesics** (drugs that decrease pain perception) may also be necessary. Narcotic analgesics (habit-forming) are usually necessary to alleviate severe pain, such as immediately after surgery. Other therapies to prevent or alleviate pain include **transcutaneous electrical nerve stimulation** (TENS) (transmits an electrical current through the skin near the point of pain), **local anesthesia, biofeedback** (allows a person to control his body functions), **epidural pain control** (injection of anesthetic into the spinal cord), surgical intervention (removal of nerve), **acupuncture** (insertion of needles at selected skin locations), and **acupressure** (application of pressure at selected acupuncture points).

Assessments to insure a person's **safety** include determination of environmental hazards that may cause injury (e.g., litter, flammable materials, poor lighting, lack of ID band, repeated exposure to X-rays, electrical equipment, bed left in high position). The presence of sensory deficits or developmental incapabilities may also predispose a person to injury.

Nursing diagnoses that pertain to safety include the following:

- Violence, potential for
- Trauma, potential for
- Suffocation, potential for
- Poisoning, potential for
- Injury: potential for

Planning and implementation strategies to prevent injury include maintenance of a safe environment, the reporting of faulty medical devices, the provision of thorough explanations, and measures to prevent falls (the elderly are especially prone).

Restraints are appropriate for use with a person at risk for hurting himself or herself or others. Documentation of the need for the restraint and the person's response to the restraint is imperative. Restraints should be checked frequently and the skin beneath the restraint checked for breakdown or problems with circulation at least every two hours. Movement and position changes should be continued.

Fire safety involves identification of factors that create the potential for fire (flammable or combustible liquids or gases such as oxygen, smoking, electricity hazards) and education regarding the location of fire extinguisher, evacuation plans, and the means to notify appropriate persons in the event of a fire. If a fire does start, client safety is maintained by calling for help immediately, removing the person from the burning area, and extinguishing the flames with a fire extinguisher. A person on fire should be rolled on the floor to extinguish flames. To prevent inhalation of smoke, crawling along the floor is advocated. Elevators should not be used. Predetermined evacuation routes should be followed.

DRILL AND PRACTICE QUESTIONS FOR REVIEW

Complete the statements below.

1. When making a bed of a client who requires frequent position changes, a _____ sheet should be used.

2. A closed unoccupied bed should be left in the _____ position. A surgical bed should be left in the _____ position.

3. When making an occupied bed, client safety is maintained by keeping the far siderail in the _____ position.

4. A person experiencing pain would probably exhibit an increase in _____, _____, and _____.

5. The most common cause of death in newborns is _____.

6. Before administering morphine to a person in pain, the _____ should be checked to make sure it is over _____.

7. An environment with high humidity can be corrected with the use of an _____.

8. A nurse massages the back of a person with back pain. The patient experiences relief of discomfort. It is likely that the backrub stimulates _____ nerve fibers.

9. A patient in pain becomes nauseous and feels faint. His pain would be described as _____.

10. When describing pain that comes and goes, the nurse should use the word _____.

11. When a nurse bathes a person in pain and tells the person that the bath will help her feel better, the nurse is using the _____ effect.

12. Biofeedback is useful in promoting alpha waves, which accompany _____.

13. The use of _____ for pain relief involves the insertion of needles in selected skin locations.

14. Newborns who require specialized care and an increased environmental temperature are placed in an _____.

15. A disoriented client is best restrained in a wheelchair with the use of a _____ restraint.

16. To restrain an infant during a procedure, a _____ restraint should be used.

Determine whether the following statements are TRUE or FALSE.

1. Caution should be exercised when using electrical equipment with a frayed cord.

2. Patient identification is best obtained by having the person tell you his or her name.

3. To prevent infection in a person with an open cut, clean techniques should be used.

4. Analgesics should be administered immediately after a painful procedure is begun.

5. A person receiving an analgesic is more prone to injury because his ability to feel sensations in general is lessened.

6. An inactivate person requires an environmental temperature higher than an active person requires.

7. In general, postop patients should not be given habit-forming narcotics for alleviation of pain.

8. In general, higher anxiety levels are associated with increased pain perception.

9. Because of the potential for drug addiction, persons in pain should not be permitted to control their own relief with narcotics.

10. Persons in acute pain should be kept busy and more physically active than usual.

11. Responses to pain vary from person to person.

12. In general, clients who use TENS postop require less pain medication.

13. When making a bed, linen should be shook free of large pieces of lint that could irritate the clients' skin.

14. The bed should be kept in the low position when changing the linen of an unoccupied bed to provide for safety.

15. When exiting a smoke-filled room, a person should crouch near the floor.

Situation

A preop client has agreed to use TENS for pain relief postop. Preoperative teaching will include a discussion of guidelines for use of TENS. Mention points that should be addressed.

ANSWERS TO DRILL AND PRACTICE QUESTIONS

Completion Exercises

1. draw

2. low, high

3. raised

4. P, R, BP

5. aspiration

6. respiratory rate, 16

7. air conditioner

8. large

9. severe

10. intermittent

11. placebo

12. relaxation

13. acupuncture

14. isolette

15. body

16. mummy

True/False Exercises

1.	F	8.	T
2.	F	9.	F
3.	F	10.	F
4.	F	11.	T
5.	T	12.	T
6.	T	13.	F
7.	F	14.	F
		15.	T

Situation

Guidelines for use of TENS:

- the activation unit should be removed for bathing or showering
- the cord should be located in such a way to avoid pulling at the skin electrodes with movement
- the activation unit should be kept away from areas of potential moisture
- the activation unit may be kept attached to the siderail
- the nurse should be alerted if an electrode dislodges
- the unit should be activated by the client as necessary (pain anticipated or actual)
- pain medication is still available as necessary

Chapter 35

REST AND SLEEP

NOTE TO STUDENT

Make sure you review the methods of providing for rest that are summarized in the table in Chapter 35.

MAJOR NURSING CONCEPTS

A period of quiet activity is called **rest,** while **sleep** refers to periodic intervals of diminished consciousness. Both serve to refresh and restore physical and mental well-being.

Physical rest often occurs naturally during each day, such as when one sits. **sitting** reduces muscle workload, lowers blood pressure, and decreases the workload of the heart. **Mental rest,** provided by enjoyable non-stress-related activities, reduces anxiety levels and improves problem-solving abilities.

One's **sleep-wake patterns** are affected by one's biorhythm called the **circadian rhythm** (cycle that repeats approximately every twenty-four hours). Circadian rhythms are established at about three months of age and determine if a person is most wide-awake in the morning, afternoon, or evening.

Other biological rhythms include **infradian** (monthly) rhythms and **ultradian** (cycle repeats in less than twenty-four hours) rhythms.

The **process of sleep** is composed of **repeated cycles** averaging ninety minutes each. Each cycle consists of five distinct **stages.** The first four stages are called **NREM (non rapid eye movement)** stages I-IV. During each consecutive NREM stage of sleep, the person experiences deepening levels of sleep accompanied by progressive decreases in heart rate, respiratory rate, systolic blood, falling basal metabolism rate, and skeletal muscle relaxation. Stage IV NREM is termed **essential** sleep. However, all the NREM stages are referred to as **obligatory** sleep because they are necessary for the healthy restoration of the body. **REM** sleep, which is the fifth stage, is called paradoxical sleep because the person appears active even though he or she is very sound asleep. Rapid eye movements, an increased and irregular respiratory rate, body movements, and penile erections characterize this stage. REM sleep is thought to coordinate binocular vision, release tensions, and provide a fail-safe measure preventing vital signs from decreasing too low.

A **nursing assessment** should ascertain **nighttime rituals** (reading, snacks, back rub, lighting), use of sleep medication, and symptoms of sleep deprivation such as irritability, and poor problem-solving ability.

159

Sleep pattern disturbance is one diagnosis accepted by the North American Association of Nursing Diagnoses.

Nursing interventions appropriate for sleep promotion include **providing comfort,** such as smooth sheets and backrubs; **hygiene measures,** such as brushing teeth and washing hands and face; **anxiety reduction;** and **pain relief** measures.

A **newborn** should be placed in the side-lying or prone position for sleep, without a pillow, and on a firm mattress for back support. Newborns sleep about sixteen hours a day and awake every four hours because of thirst.

Infants either sleep or are active during the first six months. However, after six months they may enjoy a short afternoon rest time. At approximately four months, an infant sleeps fifteen hours a day. Babies who have been given bottles propped in bed in order to induce sleep often develop extensive dental cavities.

Toddlers sleep ten to fourteen hours each day, which usually includes an afternoon nap. Bedtime rituals are very important to the toddler. Bedtime rituals should be recognized and integrated into the nursing care plan if the toddler is admitted to a health-care facility.

Many **preschoolers** abandon the afternoon nap. Because they are almost universally **afraid of the dark,** sleep promotion interventions for the preschooler should include use of a night light.

The **school-ager** has needs for mental rest as well as physical rest and sleep. Sleep disturbance in older school-age children may occur because they are worrying about grades or about their physical appearance.

Because of their often hectic schedules and significant growth spurts, **adolescents** require much sleep as well as mental and physical rest periods. Few adolescents are aware of these needs, and instead, attempt to stay up late in an effort to declare their independence and maturity.

Young adults may develop problems with sleep because of anxiety from work pressures. Pregnant women need to reserve time each day for rest periods. Many young adults experience sleep deprivation because of an infant's wakefulness or because of a sick child.

The career-oriented, **middle-aged adult** often needs to be reminded of the importance of daily rest periods (may be in the form of exercise for those with desk jobs). Tenseness and anxiety may produce sleep disturbance, especially for adults who work variable shifts, necessitating the routine use of sleep medications.

The **older adult** may experience **insomnia** (inability to sleep at night) because of cat-napping during the day or because of lack of stimulation and activity which produce healthy fatigue. The older adult, however, requires only six hours of sleep each night.

Persons with **respiratory** or **cardiac conditions** tire more quickly than others and maintaining a semi-Fowler's position improves respiratory and cardiac function. Persons with **major trauma** are usually exhausted because their physical resources are spent on dealing with fear, pain, and massive healing. A lowered hemoglobin level from hemorrhage makes it difficult for the body to transport oxygen and nutrients to the cells, leading to fatigue. Treatment consists of oral iron supplements or a blood transfusion and planned periods of rest. The increased basal metabolism level caused by fever in persons with **infection** can deplete nutrient stores and causes exhaustion. Persons with infection, therefore, need more rest and nutrients.

Additional conditions which reduce energy levels are **decreased nutrient intake** (from oral surgery, head injury, depression, gastrointestinal illness), **defects in carbohydrate metabolism,** and body image change (loss of a leg, hysterectomy, pregnancy, mastectomy, or after a heart attack). Any one of these events can cause fatigue for months afterward.

Hazards of rest include complications of immobility such as increased cardiac workload, osteoporosis, urinary tract stones, urinary tract infection, and thrombophlebitis (clot and inflammation of blood vessels). Nursing measures designed to prevent these hazards are discussed in Chapter 35.

Sleep is important, and nursing interventions which promote sleep should include **environmental factors** (adequate warmth, low noise levels, dim lighting), **timing** (adhering as much as possible to the person's usual bedtime), bedtime (HS) **rituals, providing sedentary activities close to bedtime, anxiety reduction** (allowing the person to verbalize, tranquilizer) and **evening care** (teethbrushing, hands and face wash, and backrub).

Medications should be given to relieve pain. However, sleep medications (**sedatives** cause mild depression of incoming stimuli, while **hypnotics** actively induce sleep) should not be the prime method of inducing sleep. People who habitually take medication to induce sleep develop tolerance to the drugs and a need for greater amounts of these medications. **Barbituates** suppress REM sleep, while chloral hydrate is a nonbarbituate hypnotic that does not suppress REM sleep. **Amphetamines** and **caffeine** interfere with sleep.

Common sleep problems include insomnia (inability to fall asleep or to remain sleeping), which is often attributed to anxiety, lack of exercise, a personality tendency to internalize emotions, and stressful life events. some people experience **myoclonic spasms** (harmless body jerks occurring as one is falling asleep) strong enough to waken them.

Involuntary urination (**enuresis**) is called **nocturnal enuresis** when it occurs at night. Nocturnal enuresis is more common in boys, the cause is unknown, and children eventually outgrow it. Some children experience **night terrors** (frightening and realistic dreams) soon after falling asleep. Night terrors experienced by adults are treated with **imipramine.**

Somnambulism is sleepwalking. Sleepwalking is sometimes frightening, and is dangerous in the hospital setting. Sleepwalkers should be awakened gently, reoriented, and returned to bed. **Sleeptalking** occurs during REM sleep and is harmless.

Narcolepsy (irrepressible need to sleep during the day) is treated with drugs which cause wakefulness such as caffeine, Ritalin, and Dexedrine.

Sleep apnea in the adult refers to oxygen deprivation during sleep due to laryngeal relaxation. Adults unconsciously respond by forcing air against the larnyx and then taking several deep breaths. Sleep apnea in infants occurs most often in the premature, may be fatal, and is considered the cause of sudden infant death syndrome (**SIDS**). Aminophylline is used to treat sleep apnea in infants.

Sleep deprivation results in disorientation, misperceptions, irritability, feelings of persecution, and marked physical fatigue. Loss of REM sleep causes anxiety, inability to deal with stress, increased appetite, and irritability. Apathy and depression are consequences of loss of NREM sleep.

DRILL AND PRACTICE QUESTIONS

Complete the statements below.

1. A time of reduced consciousness that restores physical and mental well-being is called _____.

2. A period of quiet activity that promotes a sense of feeling refreshed is called _____.

3. The term _____ refers to internal rhythm systems that affect body functions such as the sleep-wake pattern.

4. The specific biorhythm which affects the sleep-wake pattern is called a _____ rhythm.

5. Rest periods are needed throughout the day for _____ and _____ rejuvenation.

6. While sitting, a person's blood pressure is _____.

7. Eighty percent of a person's sleep time is occupied by _____ type of sleep.

8. Irregular respirations, blood pressure fluctuations, and rapid eye movements are characteristics of _____ type of sleep.

9. NREM sleep is termed _____ sleep because its purpose seems to be rest and restoration of the body.

10. A sleep-related nursing diagnosis accepted by the North American Association of Nursing Diagnoses is _____.

11. The safest positions for babies to sleep in are the _____ and the _____ positions.

12. Toddlers often depend on familiar routines each night when preparing for sleep. These routines are called _____.

13. Persons with cardiorespiratory illnesses prefer to sleep in the _____ position.

14. The excessive use of the bed rest can result in _____, _____, _____, and _____.

15. A _____ is a medication which helps a person to fall asleep by decreasing incoming stimuli.

16. A medication which actively induces sleep is called a _____.

17. Involuntary body jerks occurring as a person begins to fall asleep are referred to as _____.

18. Somnambulism is _____.

19. A neurological disorder resulting in an uncontrollable need for sleep is called _____.

20. The cause of SIDS (sudden infant death syndrome) is often related to _____.

Determine whether the following statements are TRUE or FALSE.

1. There are few differences among people in their need for sleep and rest.

2. A person's biorhythms may have been influenced by the mother's biorhythms while still in utero.

3. Periods of sitting or lying down provide essential physical rest.

4. Stress and anxiety often interfere with sleep.

5. Sleeping may be some people's method of dealing with stress.

6. REM sleep is essential for physical and mental rejuvenation, but NREM sleep is not essential.

7. NREM sleep is called paradoxical sleep because during this time, the body appears active.

8. Nurses need not assess an adult's normal bedtime rituals but should carefully assess a child's bedtime rituals.

9. Nurses should be aware that bright lights, noise, and the unfamiliar surrounds in the hospital setting interfere with sleep.

10. Daytime napping may interfere with sleeping at night.

11. Relieving pain and providing comfort measures are important nursing interventions int he promotion of sleep.

12. Nurses should teach parents of infants that propping a bottle in the bed is an effective method of helping the baby fall asleep.

13. Most newborns awake every four hours because they are thirsty.

14. Preschoolers often need nightlights because of their fear of the dark.

15. Adolescents need less sleep than the school-age child.

16. In order to improve an older adult's sleeping patterns, the nurse should recommend an increase in activity.

17. Pain and fear contribute to exhaustion in the person who has experienced a major trauma.

18. The nurse needs to be aware that body temperatures fall during sleep.

19. When caring for a client with insomnia, the nurse's first response should be to offer a sleeping medication.

20. Nocturnal enuresis is caused by congenitally weakened bladder tone.

Situation

Mr. Jenkins is a forty-six-year-old accountant who comes to the HMO where you work because of a mild eye infection. He tells the nurse that his only other complaint is insomnia. The nurse ascertains information from Mr. Jenkins about his six day a week, twelve hour working day, his job related stress, anxiety over his teenage son's falling school grades, his increasing alcohol consumption, and his lack of exercise. This nurse writes a care plan for Mr. Jenkins specifically designed to promote sleep and rest. List several nursing interventions you would incorporate into this care plan.

ANSWERS TO DRILL AND PRACTICE QUESTIONS

Completion Exercises

1. sleep
2. rest
3. biorhythms
4. circadian
5. mental, physical
6. reduced (or decreased)
7. NREM
8. REM
9. mandatory (or obligatory)
10. sleep pattern disturbance
11. side-lying, prone
12. bedtime rituals
13. semi-fowlers
14. osteoporosis, kidney stones, urinary tract infections, thrombophlebitis
15. sedative
16. hypnotic
17. myoclonic spasm
18. sleepwalking
19. narcolepsy
20. sleep apnea

True/False Exercises

1. F
2. T
3. T
4. T
5. T
6. F
7. T
8. D
9. T
10. T
11. T
12. F
13. T
14. T
15. F
16. T
17. T
18. T
19. F
20. F

Incorporate rest periods throughout the day.

Start a daily exercise program (taking a leisurely walk, for example).

Reduce alcohol consumption.

Avoid caffeine after lunch.

Give Mr. Jenkins a list of foods containing caffeine (coffee, tea, cola, chocolate).

Avoid stimulating activities close to bedtime; plan some type of quiet activity before bedtime.

Take time to practice bedtime rituals such as brushing teeth, washing hands and face, reading, drinking a glass of milk.

Ask the family's assistance in providing a quiet, dimly lit environment.

Avoid any daytime napping.

Teach Mr. Jenkins anxiety reduction techniques such as relaxation therapy.

Give Mr. Jenkins complete and thorough information about his eye infection, its treatment, and expected outcomes in order to decrease anxiety levels.

Chapter 36

NUTRITION IN HEALTH

NOTE TO STUDENT

Be sure to review Tables 36-3 (foods from each of the five food groups), 36-4 (functions of required nutrients), 36-6 (sources and functions of minerals), and 36-7 (vitamins).

MAJOR NURSING CONCEPTS

Normal nutrition is necessary for growth, energy, hormonal function, resistance against infection, and emotional well-being. Poor nutritional states can be **primary** (diet is deficient) or **secondary** (some body process is abnormal, interfering with ingestion, digestion, transport, and/or utilization of nutrients). **Undernutrition** occurs when a person's diet is insufficient in nutrient quantity, while **malnutrition** occurs when a diet is deficient in the quality of nutrients it includes. **Overnutrition** occurs when a diet is excessive in the amount of nutrients it includes.

The amount of nutrients required for each person per day depends on his/her **basal metabolic rate,** or BMR (minimum amount of energy needed for routine body processes), and individual activity and growth needs. Ingested nutrients are utilized for body processes or energy or stored for later breakdown (**catabolism**) and use. Extra nutrients are required in times of stress or trauma, when energy demands are increased or **anabolic** (tissue building) processes are required.

Nutrients necessary for cell growth and function include carbohydrates, protein, fat, minerals, vitamins, and water. Recommended daily allowances (RDA) for kilocalories (represent energy found in food), protein, and certain vitamins and minerals have been established. Consumption of a diet that includes foods from five food groups (fats, meats, dairy products, breads and cereals, fruits and vegetables) should help insure that a person is consuming all necessary nutrients in adequate amounts.

Carbohydrates are necessary to provide energy for cell function. Carbohydrates can be used immediately or stored as fat or glycogen for later use. They are inexpensive sources of calories. **Insulin** (absent or deficient in diabetes) is necessary for use of carbohydrates by cells. Inappropriate intake and/or utilization of carbohydrates can cause dental caries, night bottle syndrome (tooth decay infants), lactose intolerance (inability to digest the sugar in milk and milk products), or obesity. Obesity predisposes a person to heart disease, stroke, hypertension, and diabetes.

Proteins, in the form of amino acids, are necessary for cell growth and maintenance, the manufacture of enzymes, hormones, and antibodies, and maintenance of body fluid balance and pH. In the absence of carbohydrate, they can also be broken down for energy, resulting in muscle wasting. Animal sources tend to provide **complete proteins** (contain all the essential amino acids), while vegetable and plant sources usually provide **incomplete proteins.** Sources of complete and incomplete proteins can be combined in the diet to provide all **essential amino acids** (those that must be taken in the diet). Adequate intake of protein is necessary to prevent

166

a **negative nitrogen balance** (catabolism exceeds anabolism). In the absence of carbohydrates, protein may be used to provide energy, precipitating a negative nitrogen balance. Protein malnutrition may cause kwashiorkor (moderate protein deficiency) or marasmus (extreme protein and/or calorie deficiency). Protein-rich foods are expensive.

Lipids (fats and oils) are important for cell structure, the transport of fat-soluble vitamins, a reserve supply of energy (when carbohydrates and protein are unavailable), and insulation of body structures. When lipids are utilized for energy, the body can become acidic, and cell metabolism and function impaired. Lipids are a more concentrated source of kilocalories than carbohydrates or protein. **Saturated fats** (animal sources, egg yolk, liver), in contrast to **unsaturated fats** (plant and vegetable sources) increase cholesterol levels in the blood stream and can cause **atherosclerosis** (narrowing of the arteries and interference with circulation). A high fiber diet consisting of unsaturated fats, and daily exercise, can help to keep serum cholesterol levels in the normal range.

There are many required minerals. **Calcium** is required for normal development and function of bones and teeth and for normal muscle function, as is **magnesium.** Decreased intake or absorption of calcium (due to lack of Vitamin D and/or stomach acidity) can cause **rickets** in children and **osteomalacia** or **osteoporosis** in adults (brittle, malformed bones). **Tetany** (generalized muscle spasms) can also occur when total body calcium levels are decreased. **Sodium** and **chloride** are responsible for normal fluid balance in the body. Excessive intake can cause hypertension. **Potassium** is necessary for normal function of muscles (including the heart). Excessive perspiration or the use of diuretics can precipitate low levels of potassium, causing muscle weakness and heart problems. **Sulfur** is responsible for the normal utilization of glucose and the structure of proteins. **Iodine** is necessary for normal function of the thyroid gland, which regulates BMR and all cell metabolism. **Iron** is necessary for normal oxygenation of cells; patients with iron-deficiency anemia (a major health problem) have a low hemoglobin and hematocrit and become easily fatigued. Iron-rich foods, such as meats, are expensive.

Other required nutrients include the water-soluble and fat-soluble vitamins (A,D,E,K). Fat-soluble vitamins can be stored in the body; and toxicity can occur if too much of a fat-soluble vitamin is consumed. Water-soluble vitamins are not stored well in the body and must be continuously consumed in the diet to maintain required levels.

Assessment of a person's usual nutritional intake can be accomplished by obtaining a **twenty-four-hour recall history** of food intake and comparing the quantity and types of foods consumed with those that are recommended. Knowledge of good nutrition should be determined. History and physical assessment findings (especially height and weight when compared to growth charts and tables of ideal weight) are also important in assessing nutritional status.

Specific **nursing diagnoses** related to nutritional status include the following:

- Nutrition, alteration in: less than body requirements
- Nutrition, alteration in: more than body requirements
- Nutrition, alteration in: potential for more than body requirements

When **planning** and **implementing** care for persons with actual or potential nutritional problems, the meaning of food to them and their lifestyles, religion, culture, finances, customs, habits, and personal desires must be considered. Stress tends to make people alter the amount of food they consume (increase or decrease).

Nutritional requirements vary with age and BMR. **Pregnant and breast-feeding women** require additional calories and nutrients (especially protein, iron, calcium, magnesium, and phosphorus). **Newborns** require more calories per pound of body weight than any other age group because of their high BMR. Breast milk, in contrast to commercial formulas, provides

167

a newborn with antibody protection against infection and is more easily digested. Soft foods, introduced individually, are started at four to six months of age to insure RDA recommendations are met in an **infant.** By one year, an infant can begin consumption of milk instead of formula or breast milk. Excessive milk intake, as a substitution for other foods, can cause obesity and deficiency states (e.g., protein, iron). **Toddlers** are capable of feeding themselves, especially finger foods, although a decreased appetite is expected, as growth slows. During the **preschool period,** growth is also slow, and appetite is decreased. Nutritious snacks are especially important during these years. **School-age children** are strongly influenced by peers. Poor food choices may be responsible for obesity, especially in boys. A nutritious diet and adequate activity are imperative in prevention of obesity at this stage. **Adolescents** experience periods of rapid growth, and require increased calories and nutrients (especially iron, calcium, folic acid, vitamin A). Participation in sports requires extra intake of calories and carbohydrates, although glycogen-loading and consumption of a high-fat diet are not recommended. Fad diets and chronic dieting should be discouraged. The conditions **anorexia nervosa**(extreme weight loss and aversion to food) and **bulimia** (bingelike overeating) may occur in adolescents, especially girls who are concerned about the attractiveness of their body size.

Young adults generally have a good appetite, although lack of knowledge of good nutrition or poor finances can contribute to poor nutritional status. **Middle-aged adults** may eat too many "fast-foods," consume an unhealthy amount of alcohol, and/or neglect their nutritional health in general. **Cholelithiasis** (gallstones) or **cholecystitis** (inflammation of the gallbladder) may cause pain after ingestion of fatty foods. Males are at particular risk for **hypercholesterolemia** and should be advised to restrict their intake of cholesterol in their diet. **Older adults** may experience a diminished appetite. Fewer calories are required as activity diminishes, but all the required nutrients must continue to be consumed. Osteoporosis may occur, and calcium is still necessary to reverse its effects. Consumption of fiber in the diet is especially important in preventing constipation. Loneliness and poor finances may contribute to nutritional deficiencies. Community services (such as Meals-on-Wheels) may be instrumental in facilitating better nutrition.

Nutritional counseling can be provided by the nurse or a **dietician.** Referral to a visiting nurse service for nutritional counseling may be necessary for patients being discharged from acute care facilities. People can be taught to read food labels to determine nutrient and caloric content.

DRILL AND PRACTICE QUESTIONS FOR REVIEW

Complete the statements below.

1. In comparison to school-age children, the appetite of toddlers and preschoolers is usually _____.

2. When a person's diet is adequate in amount of food but deficient in specific nutrients, the person is said to be _____.

3. The energy found in food is measured in _____.

4. The nutrient that is the body's preferred source of energy is _____. When this nutrient is not available, _____ and _____ can be used for energy.

5. The form of carbohydrate that supplies energy to cells is _____. The hormone necessary for utilization of this carbohydrate form is _____.

6. When a person's body is involved in more breakdown than buildup of protein, the person is said to be in a _____ balance.

7. The five food groups include _____, _____, _____, _____, and _____.

8. The forms of carbohydrate that are especially important in the maintenance of bowel tone are _____ and _____.

9. Lack of glucose is especially damaging to _____ cells.

10. If fats are broken down to provide energy for cells, the pH of body fluids may become abnormal. Specifically, body fluids may become more _____ than normal.

11. To prevent dental caries, people can be taught to drink water and use toothpaste that contain _____.

12. Obesity is thought to predispose people to _____, _____, _____, and _____.

13. To facilitate postoperative tissue healing, the nutrient, _____, should be increased in the diet.

14. A child who consumes a low-protein diet develops swelling of the abdomen and fails to gain weight. This condition is called _____.

15. To prevent atherosclerosis, a diet low in _____ fats should be consumed.

16. Menstruating adolescents should be advised to consume an increased amount of the mineral, _____, in their diet.

17. Persons who consume an excess amount of salt in their diet are especially predisposed to _____ blood pressure because fluid is _____.

18. A person with a goiter should be assessed for a/an _____ deficiency.

19. A person has difficulty with the clotting of his blood. A vitamin _____ deficiency should be considered as a related factor.

20. The religious belief that advocates fasting from meat on Fridays during the Lenten season is _____.

Determine whether the following statements are TRUE or FALSE.

1. The BMR of elderly persons is greater than that of middle-aged adults.

2. To prevent malnourishment in infants from low socioeconomic groups, mothers should be advised to put their infants to bed with a full bottle of formula.

3. A person who weighs 10 percent more than the normal weight of persons of the same height is said to be obese.

4. Persons who are obese as children generally have greater difficulty losing weight in later life.

5. Persons with atherosclerosis should be advised to increase their consumption of red meats.

6. A person with atherosclerosis should be advised to use hydrogenated oils for cooking.

7. Calcium deficiency may cause bones to become brittle and fracture easily.

8. People on low-salt diets should be advised to eat preserved rather than fresh meats.

9. Formula-feeding of newborns should be discouraged.

10. Adolescents with anorexia nervosa or bulimia require psychological counseling.

Match each of the following nutrients from Column A with its corresponding function from Column B. Choices from Column B can be used more than once.

Column A
1. Vitamin A
2. Vitamin D
3. Calcium
4. Vitamin K
5. Protein
6. Glucose
7. Vitamin C
8. Vitamin B12
9. Potassium
10. Vitamin E

Column B
a. regulation of calcium and phosphorus levels in the body
b provides structure to bones and teeth
c. normal corneal growth and eyesight
d. formation of factors important for blood coagulation
e. provides energy for cell function
f. prevention of pernicious anemia
g. protects fat in the body from destruction by oxygen
h. regulation of muscle function
i. muscle growth and maintenance
j. collagen formation

Situation

You are a nurse working in an acute care facility. You have just admitted June Smith, a patient scheduled for surgery, to your unit. State assessments that will be incorporated into your health assessment (history-taking and physical examination) to determine June's nutritional status. State physical assessment findings that would be considered normal.

ANSWERS TO DRILL AND PRACTICE QUESTIONS

Completion Questions

1. less

2. malnourished

3. kilocalories

4. carbohydrate, fat, protein

5. glucose, insulin

6. negative nitrogen

7. fats, breads and cereals, fruits and vegetables, dairy products, meats

8. cellulose, pectin

9. brain

10. acid

11. fluoride

12. heart disease, stroke, hypertension, diabetes

13. protein

14. kwashiorkor

15. saturated

16. iron

17. high, retained

18. iodine

19. K

20. Roman Catholic

True/False Questions

1.	F	6.	F
2.	F	7.	T
3.	F	8.	F
4.	T	9.	F
5.	F	10.	T

Matching

1.	c	6.	e
2.	a	7.	j
3.	b	8.	f
4.	d	9.	h
5.	i	10.	g

Situation

History:

- 24-hour recall history of foods consumed
- problems with nutrition, eating
- food preferences
- appetite

Physical assessment:

- height, weight
- condition of hair (shiny and strong, with good body)
- condition of eyes (moist, pink conjunctiva; good eyesight)
- condition of mouth (moist and pink mucous membranes; nontender tongue; no cavities, inflamed gingiva, cracks, or fissures)
- neck (normal contour of thyroid)
- skin (smooth, normally colored skin with normal turgor; no ecchymosis or petechiae)
- extremities (normal muscle mass, strength, and reflexes)
- finger and toenails (smooth and pink)

Chapter 37

MODIFICATIONS IN NUTRITION

NOTE TO STUDENT

Study the table that discusses Measures to Prevent Complications of TPN.

MAJOR NURSING CONCEPTS

Nursing **assessments** aimed at determining a client's nutritional status include data obtained from a **health history** (client's usual intake), and a **physical exam** (oral cavity, bowel sounds, motor coordination, sensory ability, condition of skin, hair, and nails, and anthropometric measurements). **Anthropometric measurements** include height and weight, head circumference (in children under two years of age, reflects nutrition in utero), chest circumference (may reflect muscle wasting secondary to poor nutrition), abdominal circumference, upper arm circumference (reflects amount of muscle), and skinfold thickness (reflects amount of fat in subcutaneous tissue). **Laboratory tests** and **intake and output** measurements are also helpful in determining nutritional status.

Nursing diagnoses relative to nutritional status include the following:

- Nutrition, alteration in, less than body requirements
- Nutrition, alteration in, more than body requirements
- Nutrition, alteration in, potential for more than body requirements

Planning and implementation strategies aimed at preventing nutritional problems and maintaining nutritional status include motivating people to improve their diet as necessary (helping them see how a change will help them), recognizing that dietary patterns may be influenced by cultural or religious practices, insuring that recommended foods are available, setting realistic nutritional patterns, providing food preferences, considering the physical limitations of clients when meal planning, and providing positive reinforcement when proper nutrition is followed.

A diet is prescribed for a client by a physician. Generally, a nurse can alter the consistency, but not the content of the diet, without a physician's order. **Therapeutic diets** include the **soft diet** (low residue foods for easy digestion), **bland diet** (soft, nonirritating diet for the client with ulcers), **pureed diet** (processed food for persons with difficulty chewing), and **liquid diet** (full or clear for persons with limited digestive ability). **Mineral-restricted diets** include diets that restrict sodium (cardiac disease), potassium (kidney disease), calcium (kidney or bladder stones). A **protein-restricted diet** is often ordered for persons with kidney disease. A **carbohydrate-restricted diet** is prescribed for persons with diabetes. **Fat-restricted diets** are prescribed for persons with cystic fibrosis and hypercholesterolemia. **Additive diets** include diets which include additional protein or minerals. These diets often require persons to take extra snacks.

172

Factors that interfere with normal nutrition include **anorexia** (loss of appetite), **nausea, vomiting** (regurgitation of food from the GI tract), **lack of bowel tone and bowel sounds** (e.g., secondary to immobility, surgery, anesthesia), **inadequate swallowing or gag reflex** (e.g., secondary to anesthesia), **difficulty chewing and/or swallowing, motor dysfunction** (difficulty getting food and/or feeding self) **sensory disturbances** (loss of taste, inability to see) and **respiratory distress** (creates fatigue with eating).

People on bedrest generally have a diminished appetite. Adequate nutrition can be maintained by providing small, frequent feedings, insuring that food is tasty and the proper temperature, reducing nausea as necessary (e.g., with the use of an antiemetic), providing an environment conducive to eating, allowing adequate time for meals, and encouraging adequate exercise.

When a person is unable to meet nutritional needs by oral intake, complete nutrition can be provided by **enteral feedings** (supply food via tube to the stomach, jejunum, or duodenum), or **total parenteral nutrition** (TPN). TPN provides total nutritional needs (except for lipids which must be administered separately by vein) and can also be used to increase weight (high protein, high carbohydrate, high calorie solutions). TPN is usually administered via a central vein. Complications include infection, hyperglycemia, fluid overload, and depression.

DRILL AND PRACTICE QUESTIONS FOR REVIEW

Complete the statements below.

1. Three methods of obtaining information about a person's dietary intake include _____, _____, and _____.

2. To determine if intestinal peristalsis is present prior to feeding a postop client, the nurse should assess _____.

3. Abdominal circumference is measured at the level of the _____.

4. The amount of body fat present in subcutaneous tissue is measured by determining _____.

5. A _____ diet would be appropriate for a person without teeth or dentures.

6. A _____-restricted diet is commonly prescribed for patients with cardiovascular disease.

7. To determine if a liquid is part of a clear liquid diet, the liquid should be _____.

8. A person on a gluten-free diet must avoid the grains _____, _____, _____, and _____.

9. A person with a high BUN would be placed on a _____-restricted diet.

10. Diabetics are usually on a diet that limits the amount of _____ ingested.

11. A listing of comparable foods that can be used by diabetics for meal planning is called an _____ list.

12. An elimination diet might be prescribed for a person with _____.

13. A person with a loss of appetite is described as _____.

14. A person who is vomiting should be placed in the _____ position to prevent _____.

15. After surgery, peristalsis may halt, creating a condition called _____.

Determine whether the following statements are TRUE or FALSE.

1. Because intake and output measurements are used to determine therapies, only nurses should record and tabulate them.

2. People on weight reduction diets should be encouraged to record their own weight losses.

3. A person who is nauseous should be offered small, frequent meals of pureed food.

4. Hyperactive bowel sounds suggest paralytic ileus.

5. To determine if a person's gag reflex is present, small amounts of food should be fed to the person and his tolerance determined.

6. A person with partial paralysis of the face should have food introduced into the nonparalyzed side of her mouth.

7. The unconscious person should be fed orally in the high-Fowler's position.

8. An antiemtic is commonly prescribed for the person who is nauseous.

9. Tube feedings can supply total nutritional needs.

10. To prevent the dumping syndrome, a person receiving an NG tube feeding should be placed in the supine position for thirty minutes after each feeding.

11. Continuous-drip tube feeding solution can hang for a maximum of twenty-four hours.

Situations

Situation 1

You are a nurse preparing to administer 200cc of tube feeding to Mr. Jones, a client who has an NG tube in place for feedings. Prior to administering the feeding, which nursing actions are indicated? Why?

Situation 2

A client is receiving TPN. State nursing interventions that are aimed at the prevention and detection of hypo-hyperglycemic reactions.

ANSWERS TO DRILL AND PRACTICE QUESTIONS

Completion Exercises

1. twenty-four hour recall history, food frequency questionnaire, daily log of intake for a week

2. bowel sounds and/or the passage of flatus

3. umbilicus

4. skinfold thickness

5. pureed

6. sodium

7. held up to the light to see if it is clear

174

8. wheat, rye, oats, barley

9. protein

10. carbohydrate

11. exchange

12. allergies

13. anorexic

14. semi-Fowler's side, or prone; aspiration

15. paralytic ileus

True/False Exercises

1.	F	6.	T
2.	T	7.	F
3.	F	8.	T
4.	F	9.	T
5.	F	10.	F
		11.	F

Situations

Situation 1

Nursing actions prior to tube feeding:

- bring tube feeding solution to room temperature (to prevent intestinal cramping from cold liquids)
- place client in elevated side-lying or Fowler's position (to prevent aspiration with feeding)
- don gloves (to prevent transmission of microbes harbored in body fluid)
- aspirate for stomach contents (to determine that tube is properly placed in the stomach)
- return aspirated contents (to prevent loss of electrolytes from the body and prevent alkalosis)
- if more than 150cc of gastric fluid is obtained, notify physician and withhold feeding

Situation 2

To prevent/detect hypo/hyperglycemic reactions:

- test urine for sugar and acetone q8h
- keep solution infusing at prescribed rate (do not slow or speed up)
- avoid stopping infusion of TPN abruptly
- observe for signs of hypoglycemia (dizziness, confusion, convulsion)
- observe for hyperglycemia (lightheadedness, confusion)

Chapter 38

ASEPSIS AND INFECTION CONTROL

NOTE TO STUDENT

Summary of common disinfectants and antiseptics are shown in Table 38-1; methods by which microorganisms spread are listed in Table 38-2; specific isolation techniques are discussed in Table 38-3; sterile gloving procedure is described in Procedure 38-4; and basic principles of medical and surgical asepsis are listed in the box in this chapter.

MAJOR NURSING CONCEPTS

Asepsis is the state of being free of pathogens or infection. **Aseptic technique** means performing procedures so that disease-causing organisms do not spread. **Medical asepsis (clean technique)** involves activities that reduce the number and transfer of organisms. **Surgical asepsis (sterile technique)** involves activities that keep an object free of all microorganisms.

The **infectious process** is the growth and spread of disease-causing microorganisms that cause healthy, human tissue to function inadequately, **Infection** may be localized (surgical incision, rectal abscess) or generalized (septicemia, chicken pox). Although the infectious process begins after the entry of the pathogen into a susceptible host, signs and symptoms may not appear for a long period of time.

The period of time between the invasion of the body by pathogens and the onset of symptoms of infection is referred to as the **incubation period.** This time interval depends on the pathogen and can extend to approximately twenty-one days (tetanus). The **prodromal period,** which extends from a few hours to a few days, begins with nonspecific symptoms (lethargy, low-grade fever) and ends with specific symptoms of a disease. Because symptoms are so vague and people are usually unaware that they are ill, infections may spread rapidly during this phase. The **illness period** is the time in which specific disease symptoms appear. Most illnesses manifest local signs and symptoms (erythema, pain, edema), as well as systemic symptoms (fever, headache, lethargy). Childhood infections may exhibit **exanthem** (skin rash) or **enanthem** (rash located on mucous membranes). The **convalescent period** is the time when symptoms begin to fade and the person regains strength and a sense of wellness.

Infection results from a chain of reactions which include existence of a disease-causing organism **pathogen);** a place for it to grow and multiply (**reservoir**); a means of exit from the reservoir (**portal of exit**); a method of transportation to a new and different site (**transmission**); a method of entering a new body site (**portal of entry**); and a **susceptible host.** Disrupting the chain of infection at the reservoir, portal of exit, transmission, or portal of entry in order to limit the spread of pathogens is a major nursing responsibility.

- **Pathogen.** Whether the organism is pathogenic depends on its virulence, numbers present, ability to live at body temperature, and ability to cause disease in humans. **Bacteria** are classified according to shape: spherical (cocci), rod-shaped (bacillus), corkscrew (spirochetes). **Gram-positive bacteria** resist decolorization by gentian violet, while **gram-negative bacteria** can be counterstained or decolorized again. Some bacteria may require oxygen for growth **(aerobic),** while others grow without oxygen **(anaerobic).** Bacteria may form spores that protect them from intense heat and drying.

- **Gram-positive cocci** include streptococci, staphylococci, and pneumococci. **Streptococci** grow primarily on the skin and nasal cavity. They may cause boils or severe infections in surgical wounds. They are of prime concern to health-care personnel because of their high resistancy to antibiotics. **Pneumococci** cause lung infections and pose a threat to individuals ill from other causes.

- **Gram-negative** cocci are usually nonpathogenic and are natural inhabitants of the upper respiratory tract. Two **pathogenic** forms are **Neisseria meningitis** (causes meningitis) and **Neisseria gonorrheae** (gonorrhea).

When **Gram-positive bacilli** (rod-shaped organisms) are spore-forming and anaerobic, they are called **clostridium.** They are very potent and can cause serious infections (gas gangrene, tetanus, and botulism). Aerobic nonspore-forming bacilli are called **coryne-bacteria** and may cause diptheria. They may also exist in a nonpathogenic state in the upper respiratory tract. Salmonella, shigella, and cholera are caused by **gram-negative bacilli. Spirochetes** (treponema pallidum causes syphilis) are considered a spiral bacteria. **Acid-fast bacteria** include the **mycobacterium tuberculosis** (responsible for tuberculosis) and the **mycobacterium leprae** (responsible for leprosy). This group of bacteria are coated with a waxy shell resistant to many antibiotics.

Antibiotics are a category of drugs that halt the growth of microorganisms by dissolving their cell wall. They are referred to as **bacteriocidal** if they kill organisms, and **bacteriostatic** if they halt the growth of bacteria. Antibiotics referred to as **broad spectrum** have the capacity to destroy gram-negative and gram-positive organisms.

- **Fungi** (small plants) are found on the surface of the skin and in the oral cavity, vagina, and gastrointestinal tract. They do not usually cause disease. They become pathogenic when the pH of the area changes (slightly acid media in the vagina becomes more alkaline) or when the client's immune system becomes depressed. Individuals on antibiotics are at high risk for fungal infection because fungi overgrow when the normal bowel flora are suppressed **(superimposed infection).**

- **Viruses,** the smallest organisms to cause disease, cannot carry on metabolic process independently, **Interferon** (protein) prevents virus development. **Protozoa** (one-celled parasites which cause malaria) and **metazoa** (multi-celled structures which cause pinworms) are organisms that live and thrive in an environmental host, often the gastrointestinal tract. **Rickettsieae** are small parasites (size of viruses) which transmit disease by insect bites (typhus).

- **Reservoir.** Reservoirs differ because organisms may be aerobic, anaerobic, or both. All organisms, however, need food and water to grow and multiply. Most organisms favor warm, dark places with a neutral or alkaline ph. A disease is considered **communicable** if it can be transmitted from one person to another; **endemic** if it is always present in the environment; **epidemic** if large numbers of people are affected and pandemic if the disease occurs throughout the world.

- **Microorganisms** may be spread by direct contact (touch); fomites (inanimate objects); vectors (insects) in food and water; or by air currents. **Sterilization** destroys all organisms on inanimate objects; **Antiseptics** (inhibit growth of organisms on skin, and **disinfectants** inhibit or destroy growth of organisms on inanimate objects.

- **Portals of entry** may be breaks in the skin or mucous membranes; entry into the gastrointestinal tract by contaminated food, or into the respiratory system by kissing.

- **Susceptible hosts** may be people with depressed immune systems or individuals who suffer from poor nutrition and chronic fatigue.

Assessment includes determination of precautions against infection based on age, general health, current drug therapy, broken skin, and immunizations.

Analysis includes a thorough understanding of microbiology and the transmission pattern of pathogenic organisms.

Planning includes establishing appropriate isolation precautions in order to limit infection. Planning ways to decrease a client's feeling of social isolation is also a nursing priority.

Concepts of infection across the life span:

- The **newborn** is born with antibodies to those diseases (passive immunity) for which the mother usually has sufficient antibodies (measles, polio, rubella, diptheria, petussis, and tetanus).

- In the **infant** the ability to produce antibodies is immature. Breast-feeding should be encouraged because it supplies antibodies. Infants have limited ability to resist infection at this age. The eustachian tube is short and more horizontal than that of an adult, leading to increased risk of middle ear infections.

- The **toddler and preschooler** interact with many people, thereby increasing their risk of infections.

- The **school-ager and adolescent** frequently contract upper respiratory infections (tonsillitis, swimmer's ear). Statistics indicate an increase in sexually transmitted diseases (gonorrhea, syphilis) and a decrease in mumps, measles, and rubella.

- The **adult** usually acquires infections by exposure to fellow workers who are ill. Most adults continue to be susceptible to tetanus because their immunizations are not kept current.

- **Older adults** are more susceptible to infections if they have not maintained their immunizations or have difficulty maintaining their health on limited finances.

Implementations to limit the spread of infections include both medical and surgical aseptic techniques. **Medical asepsis** (clean technique) includes proper handwashing and appropriate isolation techniques. **Isolation techniques** limit the spread of microorganisms from an infected person to a noninfected person. Seven categories of isolation precautions have been developed by the Centers for Disease Control (CDC). They include **respiratory enteric, drainage/secretion precautions, blood and body fluid precautions, contact, acid-fast, and strict.** The CDC does not recommend **protective isolation techniques;** however, many health-care agencies still use this technique for clients without immunological function (leukemia). Nursing responsibilities for clients requiring isolation are based on the mode of transmission of the causative organism. Effective isolation techniques begin with effective communication (everyone should be aware of the type of isolation in effect) and clearly written instructions stating the necessary precautions and ample supplies for proper protection.

Decreasing the risk of becoming a susceptible host can be affected by an intact immune system and the action of white blood cells. **Septicemia** occurs when pathogenic organisms enter the blood stream. **Antigens** (foreign organisms) stimulate the immune system—B-cell (humoral immunity) and T-cell (cellular immunity) to produce lymphocytes. B-cell lymphocytes develop into antibodies specific to the invading antigen, while T-cell lymphocytes destroy the antigen by direct contact or by the release of lymphokines. **Interferon** is an example of a lymphokine. **Immunity** is a state in which antibodies (immunoglobulines) are capable of preventing a specific disease. Antibodies formed in response to a particular antigen will be active against that particular antigen only. **Immunoglobulin levels** involved in immunity reach adult quantities at different ages (IgG at four years of age).

Active immunity (person develops antibodies to an antigen) may be naturally acquired or artificially acquired. **Passive immunity** (person is administered antibodies to protect against an antigen) may be naturally acquired or artificially acquired.

Vaccines and **antitoxins** are agents used either to immunize people against specific diseases or to cause artificially acquired active immunity or artificially acquired passive immunity.

- **Attenuated forms of vaccines** are made from live organisms that have been reduced in virulence. They will not cause active disease but will insure an effective antibody response.

- **Dead or inactivated forms of vaccines** are killed organisms because of the virulence of the organism.

- **Toxoids** are vaccines produced from the toxins of specific bacteria (diptheria).

- **Antitoxins** are antibodies for toxin-producing bacteria and are administered for passive immunity

Surgical asepsis (sterile technique) involves practices designed to limit the transmission of pathogens or to destroy pathogens. This technique is used when performing a procedure that involves broken skin. **Sterilization** is a process by which an object is made free of all microorganisms and spores; the object is then considered **sterile.** An object is **clean** if it is free of pathogenic organisms. Sterilization can be achieved by steam under pressure (autoclave); gas; cold; boiling; or ultraviolet radiation. **Sterile equipment** remains sterile only if handled correctly (sterile gloves, sterile dressings). A **sterile field** (the inside of a sterile wrapper) may be used as a sterile work area for other sterile supplies. The work area should be at waist level or higher, and it must be kept dry. The outside inch of the sterile field is considered contaminated. Commercially prepared sterile liquids (sterile water, sterile saline) are not resealable. Unused portions must be discarded.

Nosocomial infections (hospital-acquired infections) develop after the client is hospitalized. Most frequent sites for nosocomial infections are the urinary, respiratory, and gastrointestinal systems. Most frequent offender is poor handwashing technique. **Transient flora** are bacteria that can easily be washed away. **Resident flora** are difficult-to-remove bacteria that are found in crevices and folds of the skin.

Evaluation of infection precaution techniques should be done periodically, since the human and financial cost is high. **Infection control committees** are required by all hospitals seeking accreditation by JCAH and reimbursement by Medicare and Medicaid.

DRILL AND PRACTICE QUESTIONS FOR REVIEW

Completion Questions

1. _____ technique is the same as sterile technique.

2. In _____ asepsis the number of organisms present is reduced.

3. The _____ period extends from the time of nonspecific symptoms until specific illness symptoms appear.

4. Local symptoms of the infectious process include _____, _____, and _____.

5. _____ is defined as a rash on the skin.

6. The chain of infection includes the _____, _____, _____, _____, _____, and _____,

7. Breaking the chain of infection may occur at the _____, _____, _____, or _____.

8. Whether an organism is pathogenic depends on its _____, _____, _____, and _____.

10. Bacteria that grow only in the presence of oxygen are called _____.

11. _____ are pathogenic and cause strep throat.

12. _____ are found primarily on the skin and in the nasal cavity.

13. _____ are coated with a waxy shell resistant to normal destructive methods.

14. _____ antibiotics destroy both gram-positive and gram-negative organisms.

15. _____ prevents virus multiplication.

16. Three nursing actions that will break the chain of infection at the reservoir site are _____, _____, and _____.

17. To break the chain of infection at the transmission point, the nurse should _____ and _____.

18. To break the chain of infection at the portal of entry, the nurse should _____ and _____.

19. To break the chain of infection at the susceptible host, the nurse should _____ and _____.

20. Strict isolation techniques require that the nurse wear _____, _____, and _____ to render care.

21. Sterilization can be achieved by _____, _____, and _____.

True/False Questions

1. A pathogen is a disease-producing organism.

2. The inoculation period for the infectious process is the time interval between the invasion of the body by the organisms and the onset of symptoms.

3. During the prodromal period, infectious diseases may spread very rapidly.

4. Systemic symptoms related to the infectious process are fever, headache, and lethargy.

5. A rash on mucous membranes is called enanthem.

6. Most microorganisms are harmful to human beings.

7. Gram-positive and gram-negative bacteria are similar in nature.

8. Anaerobic bacteria can grow only in the presence of oxygen.

9. Antibiotics halt the growth of bacteria by destroying the cell membrane.

10. Patients should be routinely placed on antibiotic therapy at least two weeks prior to surgery.

11. Bacteriocidal agents halt the growth of bacteria.

12. Steroids decrease the inflammatory process and may mask infection.

13. A disease is considered pandemic if large numbers of people are affected.

14. Middle ear infections are frequent in young children because their esophagus is short and more horizontal than that of adults.

15. Respiratory isolation requires that patients be placed in a private room with the door closed.

16. Enteric isolation precautions are used to limit the spread of organisms transmitted by blood and body fluids.

17. Vaccines given to people exposed to a disease for which they have no antibodies proclude artificially acquired passive immunity.

18. A nosocomial infection is a hospital-acquires infection.

19. Wrappers that enclose sterile dressings should not be used as a sterile field because they may become wet.

20. The outer three inches of a sterile field is not considered sterile.

Situations

Situation 1

Bob Jensen, a heroin addict, is admitted to the hospital with Hepatitis, type B. State which type of isolation precautions is indicated, and list three specific nursing interventions pertaining to the isolation precaution chosen.

Situation 2

Twenty-year-old John was admitted to your unit after an emergency appendectomy. He is two days post-op, and his surgical wound requires a sterile dressing change using only sterile 4 x 4s and adhesive tape. List the equipment necessary to establish a sterile field, and describe how you would set one up. In addition, list the steps for putting on and removing sterile gloves.

Situation 3

Twelve-year-old Joan was admitted to your unit with chickenpox. In order to protect yourself and others, strict isolation technique is required. Describe the gowning procedure for entering and leaving a strict isolation room.

ANSWERS TO DRILL AND PRACTICE QUESTIONS

Completion Exercises

1. aseptic

2. medical

3. prodomal

4. erythema, pain, and swelling (edema)

5. exanthem

6. pathogen, reservoir, method of exit, transmission, portal of entry, and susceptible host

7. reservoir, portal of exit, transmission, or portal of entry

8. ability to cause disease, virulence, numbers present, and its ability to live at body temperature

9. spherical, rod-shaped, or corkscrew

10. aerobic

11. beta-hemolytic streptococci

12. staphylococci

13. acid-fast bacteria

14. broad-spectrum

15. interferon

16. frequent sterile dressing changes, empty waste-paper baskets, and frequent disposal of used tissues

17. wash hands between treating clients and use appropriate isolation precautions

18. protect skin integrity, use strict sterile technique when changing dressings, prepare food and medications appropriately, maintain correct isolation technique, and have patients wash their hands before eating and after using the bathroom.

19. keeping immunizations current and identifying susceptible, high-risk individuals and providing them with appropriate isolation precautions

20. mask, gown, and gloves

21. steam, gas, and cold

True/False Exercises

1.	T	11.	F
2.	F	12.	T
3.	T	13.	F
4.	T	14.	F
5.	T	15.	T
6.	F	16.	F
7.	F	17.	T
8.	F	18.	T
9.	T	19.	F
10.	F	20.	F

Situations

Situation 1

Isolation precaution: Blood and body fluid

Nursing actions:

- wear gloves when touching body fluid or blood
- wear gown if there is a possibility of soiling your own clothes
- all objects need to be double bagged
- do not recap needles

Situation 2

Equipment necessary to establish the sterile field include the following:

- sterile towel
- the wrappers that enclose the sterile 4 x 4s that will be used as a dressing
- sterile gloves

Handwashing procedes all sterile procedures. The area that is to be used as a sterile field (e.g., overbed table) must be dry and at least waist high or above. Sterile dressing wrappers must be fully unfolded if they are to be used as a sterile field. To open a sterile towel, unwrap the outer paper and lift the towel touching only its corners. Note that the outer inch of the sterile towel or the sterile dressing wrapper is considered contaminated. If using the sterile towel as a sterile field, add sterile 4 x 4s by folding the wrapper back over your hand. Drop the sterile 4 x 4s (dressing) from the height of about 6 inches. Since the adhesive tape is not sterile, it does not belong on the sterile field.

Steps for Sterile Gloving:

- wash hands thoroughly
- select proper size gloves
- open outside wrapper with the flap farthest from you first and the flap nearest to you last
- place gloves so that cuffs are toward you, with right glove to your right
- pick up right glove by the inside of the cuff with your left hand, and insert right hand into glove
- pick up left glove with gloved right hand by slipping right hand under the cuff
- flip cuffs back by touching sterile glove sides
- adjust fit

Steps for Removing Gloves:

- pinch one glove just below the level of the thumb and remove by peeling it off, touching only glove to glove
- slip ungloved hand under thumb side of other gloved hand and peel off by touching only inside of glove
- discard appropriately
- wash hands

Situation 3

Steps for Entering a Strict Isolation Room:

- wash hands thoroughly
- assemble all necessary supplies for patient care
- don mask, gown, and gloves outside patient's room
- insert watch in plastic bag if it will be needed to monitor vital signs
- close door after entering

Steps for Leaving a Strict Isolation Room:

- place linen supplies in plastic bag and close securely
- slip plastic bag into a second bag (double-bag) held by a second person outside the room
- remove disposable supplies (soiled dressings, plastic dishes) using same double-bag technique
- to remove watch, tear plastic bag and slip it onto a clean surface immediately outside the room or into the hand of another person outside the doorway
- untie waist ties of gown
- remove gloves by grasping cuffs and peeling forward over themselves and off the hands.
- discard gloves into soiled container
- wash hands and use paper towel to turn off faucets
- untie neck ties of isolation gown
- remove gown by touching the inside only and discard into linen bag inside the room; if gown is disposable, discard
- remove disposable mask and discard
- leave room by using clean paper towel to turn doorknob
- close door from outside with clean hand
- wash hands thoroughly

Chapter 39

MEDICATION ADMINISTRATION

NOTE TO STUDENT

This is a detailed and comprehensive chapter. Be sure you review the guidelines to follow before you can administer a drug safely (Figure 39-5), medication administration techniques, medication dosage calculations, and abbreviations for medication orders.

MAJOR NURSING CONCEPTS

Medication administration is an important and complex nursing responsibility. Any substance which affects a person's health or ability to function is a **drug. Medicines** are substances which improve a person's health or ability to function.

Drugs may be categorized as **OTC** (over-the-counter), which means that no physician's prescription is necessary for its purchase. **Scheduled** drugs (a classification of drugs with drug-dependent properties) and **legend** drugs can be obtained by prescription only. Nurses must account for all scheduled drugs and must adhere to strict legal guidelines.

Drugs may have several names, such as the **generic** name (original name), **official** name (how it is listed in the official drug publications), **chemical** name (chemical description of its ingredients), and the **trade** name (manufacturer's brand name). Some of the most useful **sources of drug information** include The American Hospital Formulary Service, the Physicians' Desk Reference, nursing pharmacology textbooks, package brochures, and nursing journals. It is important for nurses to become familiar with these references because it is impossible for anyone to know all there is to know about the more than 25,000 drugs available today.

The process of a drug being distributed from its point of entry in the body into the bloodstream is termed **absorption** and is influenced by the administration route, drug solubility and concentration, acid-base balance, and administration site conditions. Since medicine cannot be absorbed in its dry form, any drug is more soluble when put into a solution (oil or water). Highly concentrated drugs are absorbed more quickly than lesser concentrated drugs. Examples of local conditions adversely affecting medication absorption include factors such as poor blood supply at injection sites, loss of skin integrity at topical application sites, or diarrhea at the rectal route.

The movement of the absorbed drug through the bloodstream to the specific site of action is called **distribution** and is dependent on adequate blood volume and blood pressure. Medication distribution often occurs across the placenta. However, most drugs do not cross the "blood-brain barrier," which protects the brain from potentially dangerous substances.

Biotransformation (conjugation) is the conversion of a drug into a usable form; since it is usually accomplished by the liver, it is important for nurses to be aware if their clients' have any liver malfunction.

Drugs may **be excreted** from the body via the lungs, intestines, breast-milk, or kidneys. In order to prevent toxic drug levels, nurses should know the route of excretion of the drugs that they administer and the client's ability to excrete the drug.

A **nursing assessment** should always include detailed information about the individual's **allergies** to medications, use of recreational drugs (narcotics, alcohol, nicotine), and OTC drugs (laxatives, birth control pills, antacids, etc.). Other factors to be included in your assessment are age (older and younger clients require lower drug dosages), body size (larger than average body size requires larger than average drug dosages), and sex (a woman during the childbearing years must be careful ingesting medications if she is, or is expecting to become, pregnant). If a person is currently taking a medication, assess whether the drug is physically achieving its desired effect, such as pain relief or blood pressure reduction. Sometimes, laboratory data are necessary to determine the drug's effects (electrolye balance, for example).

Medication effects include **therapeutic** (desired effect), **local** (affects only the area where the medication is applied), **systemic** (total body effect), **side effects** (additional harmful or helpful actions other than the therapeutic effect), **toxic** (harmful effect resulting from an overdose or an excessive accumulation of medicine), **synergistic** (a harmful or helpful enhancing effect occurring when two drugs are administered together), **antagonistic** (lessening effect occurring when two drugs are given at the same time), **untoward** (undesirable but expected effect), **adverse** (unexpected and undesirable effects such as an allergic or idiosyncratic reaction), **tolerance** (when the person needs increasingly greater dosages of a drug in order to achieve the therapeutic effect), **cumulative** (accumulation of a drug in the body usually due to poor excretion of the drug), **drug interaction** (adverse effect occurring from the simultaneous administration of two or more drugs such as the incompatibility of two drugs in an intravenous solution causing an insoluble precipitate), and **drug dependence** (physical and/or psychic addiction).

Medicines for **infants** are often available in a liquid form, or may be crushed and mixed with baby food, and are given via injection only when absolutely necessary because infants have few acceptable injection sites (vastus lateralis and deltoid only). **Toddlers** have difficulty swallowing tablets or capsules, and liquid drugs are often available. **Preschoolers** need praise for their cooperation after an injection. Children five years and younger need to be restrained for injections in order to avoid needle breakage should the child suddenly move. **School-agers** and **adolescents** need explanations about the reason for the medication, and adolescents should be questioned about the use of illegal drugs, which can interfere with the prescribed drug therapy. **Older adults** often have difficulty with medication regimes because of poor eyesight, memory loss, need to take several drugs at one time, and difficulty swallowing.

In almost all instances, physicians prescribe medications and nurses administer medications. **Administration of medication** includes **drug knowledge** (classification, safe dosage, method of administration, therapeutic effect, side effects, and toxic effects), **assessing drug appropriateness, calculating the dosage and amount** (includes knowledge of metric and apothecary systems and mathematical formulas for drug computations and conversions and **preparing the drug.** Children's dosages are determined by using the manufacturer's recommended dose per pound of body weight or surface area of the child. The **five "rights"** are rules for safe medication administration and include the right drug, right dose, right route of administration, right time, and right client. Clients have the right to refuse medication.

Oral medications are economical, convenient, frequently used, and available in many forms: tablets, capsules, lozenges, powders, effervescent powders or tablets, spansules, liquids, suspensions, and syrups. Contraindications for administering oral medications include difficulty swallowing, mouth trauma, NPO status, presence of nausea and vomiting. Oral medication are administered using clean technique.

Parenteral (by injection) medications are available as liquid in a vial, single dose ampules, powder in a vial, ready mixed vials, prefilled syringes, and Tubex syringes. Administration of parenteral medications requires sterile technique, selection of an injection site appropriate to the type of injection, selection of proper needle length and diameter, and, of course, safe injection technique. Types of injections include intradermal (shallow injection into the skin), subcutaneous (between the skin and muscle mass), intramuscular (into the muscle tissue), Z-track, and intravenous (into the vein). Sites appropriate for intradermal injection are the inner aspect of the forearm and outer aspect of the upper arm. For subcutaneous injections use the vastus lateralis (anterior thigh), deltoid (upper arm), or lower abdomen. Intramuscular injection sites include the vastus lateralis, ventrogluteal, and dorsogluteal. Contraindications for parenteral injections are infection, inflammation, edema, or scar tissue at the site.

Topical medication administration is external and includes lotions, liniments, and ointments, and may be applied with tongue blades or gloved hands. Sterile technique is necessary only when there is a loss of skin integrity. Eye drops or ointments are a type of instillation medication, must be labeled "for opthalmic use," and administered using sterile technique. Nose drops and ear drops ("otic") are also considered instillations, as is the administration of medication via the rectum or vagina. Inhalation medication administration provides a local effect on respiratory membranes via a nebulizer (fine mist spray).

DRILL AND PRACTICE QUESTIONS FOR REVIEW

Complete the statements below.

1. A substance that improves a person's health is called a _____.

2. The _____ name is the original name of a drug given by the drug company that developed the drug.

3. If a nurse wanted to identify tablets brought by a client to the emergency room, the _____ would be the most appropriate source to use.

4. Drugs which have a high potential for drug dependence are termed _____ drugs.

5. The four important pharmacokinetic processes are _____, _____, _____, and _____.

6. The oral route of medication administration is also called the _____ route.

7. The physiological barrier that protects the brain and spinal cord from potentially toxic substances is the _____.

8. The desired effect from a medication is called its _____ effect.

9. Additional effects of medications, other than the desired effect, are known as _____.

10. When a person receives a beneficial effect from a noneffective drug, it is called a _____ effect.

11. An acceptable injection site in infants for intramuscular medication administration is the _____.

12. Allowing a preschool child who is receiving injections to play with a clean syringe is called _____ play.

13. Narcotic orders have a _____ day stop order.

14. Two systems of medication administration are the _____ system and the _____ system.

15. The abbreviation which means four times a day is _____.

16. When administering medications in a health-care agency, the nurse must be familiar with the _____ and _____ systems of measurement.

17. Two grains is equal to _____ milligrams.

18. A _____ is used for determining a child's surface area.

19. The basic five rights for safe medication administration are the _____, _____, _____, _____, and _____.

20. Three common sites appropriate for subcutaneous injections are the _____, _____ and _____.

21. The muscle of the anterior thigh which is used for intramuscular injections is called the _____.

22. The two anatomical landmarks to be identified in order to use the ventrogluteal site for an intramuscular injection are the _____ and _____.

23. An injection angle of _____ degrees is used for subcutaneous injections.

24. To apply ointment to a client's skin, the nurse should use a _____ or _____.

25. When administering eye drops, the nurse should allow the drop to fall on the _____.

Determine whether the following statements are TRUE or FALSE.

1. Any substance which affects a person's health status is called medicine.

2. The brand name of a drug is also referred to as the trade name.

3. Some over-the-counter drugs are also scheduled drugs.

4. Legend drugs may be obtained only with a prescription.

5. Most drugs are biotransformed in the body by the liver.

6. Most drugs are excreted from the body by the kidneys.

7. Absorption of medicine across the skin is faster than absorption across the mucous membrane.

8. Lipid-based solutions are more readily absorbed into the gastrointestinal tract than are water-based solutions.

9. Drugs are often excreted in breast milk.

10. Generalized body effects from a medication are also known as systemic effects.

11. Medicine is more readily absorbed from the gastrointestinal tract when the stomach is full.

12. The nurse should elevate the infants head when administering an oral medication to the infant.

13. The lower abdomen is an acceptable subcutaneous injection site for an infant.

14. Two-year-old children are able to swallow capsules and tablets.

15. It is a good idea to teach older adults to keep their medicine in a conspicuous place.

16. Nurses can offer simple medications such as aspirin to a client without a physician's prescription.

17. All medication must be reordered following surgery.

18. The abbreviation, BID, means twice a day.

19. The abbreviation, gtt., means one ounce.

20. Insulin is supplied in a standard strength of 100 units per iml.

21. Children's medication dosages are determined by age or weight.

22. Medication should be charted only after it has been administered.

23. The inner aspect of the forearm is an appropriate site for an intradermal injection for allergy testing.

24. When drawing two types of insulin using the double vial technique, the nurse should always draw up the long-acting insulin first.

25. Nurses should not replace the plastic sheath over the needle following an injection.

Situations

Situation 1

Mrs. Arish delivered a healthy baby girl twenty-four hours ago. At the moment her only complaint is a headache. Her physician has left an order on the chart for Aspirin gr. 10, p.o., q4h, prn. List in sequence the steps the nurse would take when administering this oral medication to Mrs. Arish.

Situation 2

Carlos, age fourteen was admitted to the hospital for treatment of leukemia. He is receiving several intravenous anticancer drugs which have the side effect of severe nausea and vomiting. Johnny's doctor has ordered a medication to relieve the nausea and vomiting. Since this medicine will be given numerous times and via the intramuscular route, list several nursing interventions designed to limit the amount of pain Johnny will experience from these injections.

ANSWERS TO DRILL AND PRACTICE QUESTIONS

Completion Exercises

1. medicine

2. generic

3. Physicians' Desk Reference

4. scheduled

5. absorption, distribution, biotransformation, excretion

6. enteral

7. blood brain barrier

8. therapeutic

9. side effects

10. placebo

11. vastus lateralis (anterior thigh)

12. therapeutic

13. three

14. stock, unit-dose

15. QID

16. metric, apothecary

17. 120

18. Nomogram

19. right drug, right dosage, right route of administration, right time, right client

20. vastus lateralis (anterior thigh), deltoid, lower abdomen

21. vastus lateralis

22. greater trochanter of the femur, anterior iliac spine

23. 35

24. tongue blade, gauze

25. lower conjunctival sac

True/False Exercises

1.	F	13.	F
2.	T	14.	F
3.	F	15	F
4.	T	16.	F
5.	T	17.	T
6.	T	18.	T
7.	F	19.	F
8.	T	20	T
9.	T	21.	F
10.	T	22.	T
11.	F	23.	T
12.	T	24.	F
		25.	T

Situations

Situation 1

Check client's record to determine if it is four hours since the aspirin was last given.

Check client's record and ask client if she has any allergies to aspirin or aspirin products.

Wash your hands.

Choose the correct medication from either a stock bottle of aspirin or a unit dose package.

Read the bottle or package label carefully for drug name, dose, and route of administration. Check this three times: as you select the package, before you pour the aspirin into the paper cup, and as you return or dispose of package.

Place the correct number of tablets into a clean paper cup

190

Assess whether client is able to swallow.

Provide client with a glass of water.

Check client's identification band.

Place client in sitting position.

Administer medication to client.

Observe client swallowing the medication.

Record medication administration.

Assess client's level of pain in one hour.

Situation 2

In order to reduce Carlos's pain from frequent injections, the nurse would do the following:

Rotate injection sites (left and right dorsogluteal, left and right ventrogluteal, and left and right vastus lateralis).

Apply ice to the injection site for a few minutes before the injection.

Use a sharp new needle.

Insert the needle and inject the medication quickly.

Remove the needle quickly.

Massage the injection site for a few minutes immediately following the injection.

When using the dorsogluteal site, position Johnny with his toes turned in.

Use psychological distractors such as conversation and deep breathing.

PART IX

MEETING SPECIFIC HEALTH CARE NEEDS

Chapter 40

PERSONAL CARE AND HYGIENE

NOTE TO STUDENT

Review the table of Common Skin Lesions provided in the chapter.

MAJOR NURSING CONCEPTS

Providing for a person's **personal hygiene** (health and cleanliness) serves to increase self-esteem, insure comfort and safety (from infection secondary to the presence of microorganisms), and offers an opportunity for therapeutic touch and mobility (e.g., ROJM to prevent such complications as contractures and thrombi). In the process of providing for personal hygiene, the nurse also has an opportunity to assess circulation (color and temperature of the skin, Homan's sign) and the condition of the skin.

The **skin** (composed of epidermis and dermis) protects inner body structures, helps maintain fluid and electrolyte balance and normal body temperature, aids in production of Vitamin D, and exerts a mild bacteriostatic action to reduce the number of microbes on the body's surface.

When providing personal care, the skin should be **assessed** for cleanliness, intactness (e.g., presence of decubiti), color (pallor, jaundice, cyanosis, erythema are abnormal), moisture, temperature (warmth suggests increased temperature and/or circulation, coolness suggests decreased temperature and/or circulation), edema (abnormal), and turgor (poor turgor associated with poor hydration). When assessing clients with regard to the skin and personal hygiene needs, the nurse also needs to determine whether a person can perform self-care or whether the person needs assistance.

A **Nursing diagnosis** pertinent to personal hygiene needs is:

- Self-care deficit.

Planning and implementation strategies aimed at meeting personal hygiene needs should be based on individual needs. **Newborns** are given sponge baths until the umbilical cord falls off. Their skin is very sensitive because of the lack of subcutaneous tissue. **Infants** are bathed in a tub, with special attention paid to the face and diaper area to prevent infection. **Toddlers and preschoolers** are bathed in a tub, but, as with infants, should not be left alone. Ecchymoses and skin excoriations are common at this age and also in the school-age years. **School-agers and adolescents** can bathe independently (with assistance as necessary). **Adolescence and pu-**

berty brings growth of hair and an increase in perspiration, requiring increased attention to maintain cleanliness and prevent infection. **Young, pregnant women** develop stretch marks (striae) on their distended abdomen. Tub baths are permitted up to a month before delivery. From **middle to older adulthood,** the skin thins and becomes less elastic, wrinkles form, and skin dries. Soap should be used sparingly; assistance may be necessary to prevent injury.

Personal care includes bathing, a backrub, and a change of clothing and linen. It may also involve bathing a person in bed, or providing for a tub bath or shower. Personal care is generally provided in the morning before eating (**A.M. care**—hands and face are cleansed); and in the evening before retiring (**P.M. care**—hands and face are cleansed); at some point during the day, a **partial bath** (face, hands, axilla, back, perineal area) or complete bath is provided.

When **bathing** a client, clean areas are washed before less clean areas, soap is used (except if a client has dry skin), water is changed frequently to keep it clean and comfortably warm (105-110 degrees F), and gloves are used whenever contact with body fluids is anticipated. Oral care (brushing twice daily), hair care (shampoo, brushing, combing), eye care, and shaving are included as necessary. Hair is assessed for **pediculosis** (head lice, identified with presence of pruritus and small, white particles on the hair shafts). Safety measures, privacy, and proper body mechanics should be practiced throughout bathing procedures.

DRILL AND PRACTICE QUESTIONS FOR REVIEW

Complete the statements below.

1. A nurse assesses a black and blue mark on the leg of a child. This is appropriately described as an _____ when documenting care.

2. Clear, watery discharge from the nose of a client is called _____.

3. When providing oral care, an _____ basin should be provided for rinsing.

4. A positive _____ sign suggests a blood clot in the leg.

5. When washing an extremity, it should be washed in a direction from _____ to _____.

6. When washing the perineal area of a female client, strokes should be made from _____ to _____.

7. To prevent excoriation from accumulation of moisture in the perineal area, _____ can be applied after cleansing.

8. When bathing a newborn, the umbilical cord can be cleansed with _____.

9. Assessments that suggest that a child has pediculosis include _____, _____, and _____.

10. Mouth care is best accomplished with a person in the _____ position.

11. _____ can be applied to the lips of a person with dry lips for relief.

12. A drug used for removal of hair is called a _____ agent.

13. Hydrogen peroxide provides a bacteriocidal action through the process of _____.

14. When bathing a client, a nurse works from _____ to _____ areas.

15. _____ should be avoided when bathing persons with dry skin.

Determine whether the following statements are TRUE or FALSE

1. To prevent damage to sensitive penile skin, the foreskin should not be retracted when providing perineal care to a male client.

2. To insure thorough cleansing, a partially paralyzed client should not be permitted to assist with his bath.

3. When giving a client a complete bath, the bed should be in the high position.

4. A client's nails should be trimmed straight across.

5. To protect the privacy of a client taking a tub bath, the door to the tub room should be locked.

6. A six-year-old child can be left alone for a tub bath.

7. Gloves should be used when providing mouth care.

8. Eyes should be cleansed from the inner to the outer canthus.

9. Contact lenses can be left in place for surgical procedures.

10. Q-tips are appropriate for use in cleansing the ear canals.

11. Hearing aids should be left on even when not in use to prevent loss of power.

12. A person with halitosis is in need of mouth care.

13. The calf of a person with a positive Homan's sign should be massaged to relieve muscle tension.

14. Medication is necessary for a person with pediculosis.

15. A nurse is responsible for checking that self-perineal care performed by a client has been satisfactorily accomplished.

Situation

A nurse plans to administer a backrub. Describe the procedure that can be followed.

ANSWERS TO DRILL AND PRACTICE QUESTIONS

Completion Exercises

1. ecchymosis
2. rhinitis
3. emesis
4. Homan's
5. distal, proximal
6. front, back
7. powder
8. 70 percent alcohol
9. scalp pruritus, scalp excoriation, nits on hair shafts
10. Fowler's

11. petroleum jelly (Vaseline)

12. depilatory

13. oxidation

14. clean, less clean

15. soap

True/False Exercises

1.	F		8.	T
2.	F		9.	F
3.	T		10.	F
4.	T		11.	F
5.	F		12.	T
6.	F		13.	F
7.	T		14.	T
			15.	T

Situation

Backrub procedure:

- place bed in high position
- provide privacy by pulling curtain or closing door
- place lotion on hands and apply to back of client's neck
- massage neck area from shoulders to hairline with small, circular motions
- massage buttocks and back area with long, upward strokes at the vertebrae and down the lateral aspects of the back
- massage area at the base of the spine and shoulder blades with small, circular motions

Chapter 41

BODY ALIGNMENT AND BODY MOVEMENT

NOTE TO STUDENT

Types of body joints and joint motion are summarized in Table 41-1 and 41-2; range of motion exercises are summarized in Table 41-3; procedures for lifting, turning, and transferring clients using principles of body mechanics are described in the chapter.

MAJOR NURSING CONCEPTS

The **human body** is composed of over 206 bones and over 600 muscles that enable it to move in a smooth, coordinated rhythm. **Immobility**—lack of movement due to injury or prescribed as treatment—has physical, social, and psychological implications. **Social immobility** (decreased interaction with others) may lead to depression, loneliness, and decreased physical activity.

Complications of immobility include the following:

- Muscular atrophy (decrease in muscle size).
- Decrease in muscle strength.
- Fibrotic stiffening of joints, making movements difficult.
- Deformities, contractures.
- Bone changes (more cells are absorbed and secreted from bone than are replaced)
- Movement of calcium and phosphorus (components of bone) into bloodstream.
- Neurological problems due to compression on nerves.
- Reduced auditory and/or tactile stimulation.
- Reduced ability to concentrate, solve problems, and remember.
- Circulatory changes—heart rate and cardiac output increase, placing added strain on heart work.
- Sluggish neurovascular response to rising from a supine position (orthostatic hypotension).
- Thrombus (blood clot that is attached loosely to a vein wall).
- Thrombophlebitis (inflammation of vein wall with accompanying blood clot). Homan's sign (pain in the calf on dorsiflexion of the foot) may indicate thrombophlebitis.
- Embolus (blood clot that has broken loose from vein wall).

- Edema (large amounts of fluid in intracellular tissue). Edema located in body parts below the level of the heart is referred to as **dependent edema.** Immobility contributes to fluid accumulation because vessels dilate, stasis occurs, pressure increases, resulting in a fluid shift.

- Decubitus ulcers (pressure sores) occur because edematous tissue breaks down easily.

- Decreased vital capacity (amount of air exhaled after maximum inspiration).

- Poor appetite which may lead to undernutrition; weight gain may occur if clients continue to eat less food, but foods consumed are high in carbohydrates or fats.

- Difficulty using crutches, wheelchair, or ambulating.

- Constipation because of low fiber diet and decreased activity

- Renal calculi (kidney stones) due to high level of calcium being lost from bones and excreted by the kidneys.

- Urinary infection due to urinary stasis; retention with overflow because bladder has lost ability to empty.

- Negative nitrogen balance because more protein is excreted than retained. Body will have difficulty with tissue repair.

Independent nursing measures to prevent the complications of immobility include the following:

- active/passive exercise program at least once a day.

- change position of clients at least every 2 hours so that there is no sustained area of pressure on joints

- proper body alignment with no sharp body angles and

- clock, calendar, book or newspaper for time orientation.

Assessment consists of looking at body alignment, effects of immobility, gait, posture, coordination, ability to do activities of daily living (dressing, feeding), use of all extremities, range of motion, and physician's orders for activity and mobility.

Activity level across the life span differs:

- Newborns have full range of joint motion.

- Infants develop from proximal to distal, and from head to toe.

- Toddlers walk with wide-based, unsteady gait.

- Preschoolers demonstrate good motor coordination.

- School-agers begin exercise and activity patterns they will use throughout their life.

- Adolescents have postural difficulties and sports injuries.

- Adults usually exercise less than adolescents.

- Older adults may suffer from osteoporosis (loss of calcium from the bones); stiffening of joints (arthritis); and loss of size in muscles (atrophy).

Body mechanics refers to using the entire body for work, using the least effort. **Center of gravity** is the point at midpelvis just anterior to the sacrum. These are the **principles of body mechanics:**

197

- The lower the center of gravity in an object, the greater its stability; the broader the base of the object, the more stable the object.
- When lifting or pulling, avoid using the muscles of the back. Instead, use muscles of upper thighs.
- Stoop to lift objects up.
- Do not lean forward when lifting low objects.
- Inhale deeply, then pull object toward self before lifting.
- When standing, have your feet 10 to 12 inches apart, abdominal muscles flat, pelvis tilted forward, and shoulders and hips at 90-degree angles to the axis of the spine.
- When sitting, the head should be erect, shoulders in straight line with hips, and feet flat on floor or on chair footrests.
- When resting, fill body hollows with pillows for support.

Range of motion exercises (isotonic exercises) may be active, active assist, passive, or passive assist. The general principles include these:

- Motions should be gentle and smooth.
- Support the joint distal to the one being exercised.
- Move joints to the point of resistance, pain, or fatigue.
- Establish a consistent pattern.

DRILL AND PRACTICE QUESTIONS FOR REVIEW

Completion Exercises

1. _____ exercises increase peripheral resistance and ventricular pressure.
2. _____ is also known as foot drop.
3. When bones become porous and lose their strength, the condition is known as _____.
4. _____ fractures can occur when clients with low bone calcium begin to ambulate.
5. Osteoporosis in women is associated with low levels of the hormone _____.
6. _____ hypotension may occur when rising too quickly from a supine position.
7. A blood clot that forms in a vein is referred to as a _____.
8. _____ refers to inflammation of the vein with an accompanying blood clot.
9. Women following childbirth, older adults, and clients on prolonged bedrest are prone to _____.
10. A thrombus that breaks away from the vein wall and travels through the circulatory system is called an _____.
11. Three nursing activities that may reduce the risk of thrombophlebitis in the immobilized client are _____, _____, and _____.
12. Pain in the calf on dorsiflexion of the foot is referred to as _____.
13. _____ is the accumulation of large amounts of fluid in the intracellular tissue.

14. Lying in a _____ position increases the work of the respiratory system.

15. _____ and _____ are two nursing activities that can loosen and move respiratory secretions.

16. Three nursing measures that may prevent urinary stasis in the bedrest client include _____, _____, and _____.

17. A _____ nitrogen balance exists when clients excrete more protein than they retain.

18. Two nursing measures that may prevent negative nitrogen balance are _____ and _____.

19. _____ are caused by continuous and sustained pressure to a body part that interferes with circulation.

20. Three bone diseases that may occur with school-age children are _____, _____, and _____.

21. When the brain has been deprived of oxygen, with resulting motor, sensory, cognitive, and vocal problems, this is referred to as a stroke or _____.

22. Three principles of body mechanics that should be used when lifting objects include _____, _____, and _____.

23. A footboard prevents _____.

24. A _____ position is a supine position with both feet and legs in stirrups.

25. The Valsalva maneuver can occur during the act of _____ or _____.

26. A three-point (swing-through) crutch gait is used when _____.

27. Three nursing measures that will assist clients with crutch-walking are _____, _____, and _____.

28. A _____ lift assists personnel in moving clients from bed to chair or chair to bed or bathtub.

True/False Exercises

1. Dependent nursing activities to prevent complications of immobility include an active exercise program and frequent body position changes.

2. Atrophy is an increase in size of muscle tissue causing it to lose strength.

3. Range of motion exercises are an example of isotonic contractions.

4. Stiffening of joints in immobilized clients begins to occur after four weeks of bedrest.

5. Osteoblastic formation refers to new bone cells which are continuously being produced.

6. A diet high in calcium is an effective way to prevent loss of calcium from the bones.

7. Compression of nerves, particularly on bony prominences, may cause problems for the immobilized client.

8. Nerve damage can occur in less than ten minutes if pressure to an area is intense.

9. Hospitalized children should not be encouraged to do homework.

10. Lying flat in bed reduces the workload of the heart and results in lower heart rate and lower cardiac output.

11. A positive Homan's sign includes redness, warmth at site, and pain in the calf on dorsiflexion of the foot.

199

12. Independent edema occurs in body parts below the level of the heart.

13. Active/passive exercises, elastic stockings, and elevation of affected body parts are nursing measures that can reduce edema.

14. Clients on bedrest should be encouraged to move their bowels on a bedpan in a supine position.

15. Kidney stones may be caused by a high level of calcium in the urine.

16. Urinary output increases when clients are kept in a supine position for long periods of time.

17. Adolescents are prone to sports injuries and postural problems.

18. Pregnant women are encouraged to walk at least one city block during the day because walking decreases arterial circulation.

19. A principle of body mechanics is that the lower the center of gravity in an object, the greater its stability.

20. Exercise promotes circulation, respiration, and good health.

21. When assisting a client who has a weak side and a strong side, to ambulate walk on the weak side.

Situations

Situation 1

Mrs. Addison is an eighty-year-old, frail (94 lbs) woman who is hospitalized for a heart condition. She is reluctant to move in bed because of pain and discomfort. She demonstrates decreased muscle strength and limited range of motion when doing range-of-motion exercises. Her skin is intact although she is beginning to show signs of pressure on her heels, sacrum, and elbows. Her physician has prescribed bedrest for the next few days. As the nurse caring for her, prepare an appropriate nursing-care plan, including the procedure for moving her up in bed. Include the rationale for each step stated in the procedure.

Situation 2

Mr. Geller needs to have his position in bed changed at least every two hours. As the nurse caring for him, describe the procedure for turning Mr. Geller from a supine position to a left side-lying position. Include the rationale for each step.

ANSWER TO DRILL AND PRACTICE QUESTIONS

Completion Exercises

1. isometic
2. plantar flexion
3. osteoporosis
4. pathological
5. estrogen
6. orthostatic/postural

7. thrombus

8. thrombophlebitis

9. thrombophlebitis

10. embolus

11. elevation of lower extremities on pillows, ROM exercises, elastic stockings

12. Homan's sign

13. edema

14. supine

15. vibrating and clapping

16. increase fluid intake, elevate head of bed, provide foods that leave acid residue

17. negative

18. exercises, well-balanced diet with vitamin supplements

19. decubitus ulcers

20. Legg-Calve'-Perthes' disease, slipped epiphysis, displacement of femur head, or scoliosis

21. cerebral vascular accident

22. bring object close, avoid using back muscles, use muscles of upper thighs, stoop to lift

23. foot drop/plantar flexion

24. lithotomy

25. moving up in bed, straining to have bowel movement

26. no weight-bearing is allowed on one foot

27. isometric exercises for upper extremities, check rubber tips of crutches for wear, and check that crutches do not rest in axilla

28. Hoyer/hydraulic

True/False Exercises

1.	F	11.	T
2.	F	12.	F
3.	T	13.	T
4.	F	14.	F
5.	T	15.	T
6.	F	16.	T
7.	T	17.	T
8.	T	18.	F
9.	F	19.	T
10.	F	20.	T
		21.	T

Situations

Situation 1

Eighty-year-old frail woman who demonstrates difficulty and complains of discomfort when moving extremities. She demonstrates reduced muscle strength and limited range of motion for her age.

Analysis:

Impaired physical mobility related to prescribed bedrest.

Goal:

Client will not develop motor complications related to prescribed bedrest.

Criteria:

Integrity of muscular skeletal system will be maintained throughout hospitalization.

Nursing Orders:

1. When positioning, keep in proper body alignment (do not use pillows under knees; avoid sharp body angles, and use footboard).

2. Monitor circulation to all extremities.

3. Maintain range-of-motion exercise schedule.

4. Provide pain medication prior to exercises of needed.

5. Provide for well-balanced diet and encourage increased fluid intake.

Procedure for moving client up in bed:

- Wash hands, identify client, and explain procedure. This process prevents spread of microorganisms, promotes client safety, and compliance.
- Bring the bed to the high position, and lower the head of the bed. By bringing the bed to the high position, the risk of back injury is reduced. A high Fowler's position forces the nurse to work against gravity.
- Have the patient grasp the siderail on the other side of the bed and bend her knees. Position yourself in a wide stance, facing the head of the bed. This is a more stable position for the caregiver.
- Place one arm under the patient's shoulders and one arm under her hips.
- Instruct the patient to push with her heels as you lift her shoulders and hips off the sheet. Help the client slide to the head of the bed. In so doing, shift your weight forward to the foot closest to the head of the bed. Shifting of weight prevents becoming unbalanced. By lifting the patient's shoulders and hips off the sheet, you prevent shearing forces (sheet burn) inhibiting blood supply to the area.

Situation 2

Procedure for turning a patient to the left side:

- Wash hands, identify patient, and explain procedure. Reduces chance of spreading microorganisms, ensures the patient safety, and encourages patient's cooperation.
- Bring bed to high position, in order to prevent muscle strain.
- Face the patient, and place one foot in front of the other.
- Move the patient to the right side of the bed by placing one arm under his shoulders and one arm under his hips. Rock your body toward your rear leg, lift and move him toward

you. This motion eases the moving of the patient across the bed. By moving the patient to the right side of the bed, you will have ample room to turn him safely to his left side.

- Cross the patient's right leg over the left; position the patient's arms across the chest; raise the siderail and walk to the left side of the bed. Placement of the arms in this manner avoids possible injury, and the siderail protects the patient from falling.
- Lower the siderail on the left side of bed. Place one hand on the patient's shoulder and one hand on his hip. Gently roll the patient toward you.
- Place support pillows as necessary and ensure proper body alignment.

Chapter 42

FLUID AND ELECTROLYTE BALANCE

NOTE TO STUDENT

Be sure to know all normal means of fluid intake and output (Table 1), and signs and symptoms of hypovolemia and hypervolemia (Table 3). Review Figure 3 to understand the phenomenon of osmotic pressure and Table 5 for findings associated with metabolic acidosis and alkalosis. Also, because administering intravenous fluids and blood transfusions are serious nursing responsibilities, be sure to review these procedures thoroughly.

MAJOR NURSING CONCEPTS

Maintaining fluid and electrolyte balance (homeostasis) and acid-base balance in the body is of utmost importance.

Fluids in the body transport cells in the blood stream, maintain blood volume, regulate temperature, remove waste materials via the urine, and are necessary for cell metabolism. The amount of fluid in the body varies with age (older people have less, and babies have more); and fluid is distributed in the body in the extracellular compartment (in the blood stream or the spaces outside of cells) and in the intracellular compartment (within the cells).

Electrolytes such as sodium, potassium, calcium, magnesium, chlorides, phosphates, and bicarbonates are substances which produce positive ions (cations) or negative ions (anions) when dissolved in water. Each of these electrolytes serve important and particular functions in the body. Normal electrolyte concentrations produce an isotonic state; high concentrations produce hypertonicity; and low concentrations produce hypotonicity.

Factors which regulate fluid volume balance and the concentration of body fluids include the principle of osmosis, hydrostatic or oncotic pressure, antidiuretic hormone production (causes fluid loss), aldosterone secretion (causes fluid retention), thyroid hormone (indirectly causes increased urine production), kidney function, and the thirst response.

Acid-base balance refers to the pH of body fluids which are usually alkaline (pH between 7.35 and 7.45). Since pH under 7.0 or over 7.8 is fatal, the body uses three buffer systems (buffer salts, respiratory excretion of carbon dioxide, and kidney excretion of hydrogen or bicarbonate ions) in an effort to maintain normal pH values.

Assessing fluid, electrolyte, and acid-base balance is an important nursing responsibility. Your health history should include questions about weight loss or gain, swelling of extremities, vomiting or diarrhea, dieting for weight loss, use of diuretic medications, and kidney disease. Physical examination should include weight determination, girth measurements (chest, waist, ankle, calf), peripheral vein emptying and filling (normal is under 3 seconds), observation of neck veins, urinary output, pulse rate, rhythm and quality (thready or bounding), respiratory rate, blood pressure, temperature, skin turgor, edema, and observation of sunken eyeballs.

Nurses should also assess laboratory data relevant to fluid and electrolyte balance such as hematocrit; urine specific gravity; and serum sodium, potassium, chloride, and magnesium levels (see Appendix G). Gastric and intestinal suctioning, hemorrhage, draining wounds, ascites (an accumulation of fluid in the abdominal cavity), stress, and anorexia nervosa are additional factors associated with imbalances in fluids, electrolytes, and acid-basis status.

Nursing diagnoses relevant to fluid and electrolyte imbalances are "fluid volume deficit" and "fluid volume excess."

Nursing interventions relevant to fluid and electrolyte imbalances include maintaining oral fluid intake requirements ("encouraging fluids") or restrictions, intravenous therapy, oral and intravenous replacement of electrolytes, recording intake and output, oral care, good skin care, elevating edematous extremities, and the application of antiemboli stockings.

Infants who are ill frequently drink less; and if the illness is complicated by diarrhea, the child is in grave danger of quickly developing a fatal fluid and electrolyte imbalance. **Toddlers** and **preschoolers** may be encouraged to take additional fluids by offering them popsicles, sherbet, or jello. Give **school-agers** and **adolescents** some control over their illness by allowing them to choose the liquids they want to drink and to keep their own intake record. The **young-adult** and **middle-aged adult** are normally cooperative about fluid regulation programs. The **older adult** may become dehydrated because of diminished kidney function and because of their fixed incomes do not allow them a choice of beverages.

Intravenous therapy replaces fluids quickly and is used in a multitude of clinical situations. The dorsal veins of the hands, forearm veins (basilic, cephalic), and veins in the inner elbow (antecubital space) are the most frequently used sites for **intravenous therapy.** Intravenous fluid is usually administered through large needles (No. 22, 20, or 18). "Butterfly" or "scalp vein" needles have an extra flange of plastic on both sides of the needle hub and are used at any site that is difficult to enter. **Intracaths** are plastic needles that theoretically will infiltrate less often because of their ability to bend. However, they may break off in the patient's vein. When removing an intracath be sure to determine if the entire needle is intact. If it is not, immediately place a tourniquet proximal to the puncture site and notify the physician.

In order to initiate intravenous therapy, a **venipuncture** must be done. This is a sterile technique done by the nurse using gloves for infection protection and a specific technique. **Intravenous fluids** are considered medications, and the physician's order should specify the type, amount, rate of infusion (except for **"Keep Vein Open"** infusions which normally infuse at 10 to 20 ml. per hour), and the specifics about additives. Intravenous fluids may be isotonic, hypotonic, or hypertonic and may be supplied in various size glass bottles or plastic bags. Various **types of tubing** are also available such as minidrip tubing, Buretrol and Solusets, Y-type tubing, and "Piggyback" set-ups. Each type of tubing has a specific drop rate (number of drops to the millimeter) which it is necessary to know in order to determine how many drops per minute the nurse will infuse the intravenous fluid. A useful **drop rate formula** is presented in the text. Most intravenous tubings contain a filter that prevents unwanted particles from entering the patient's bloodstream. Infusion-administration pumps automatically regulate the infusion rate and are helpful; however, they do not relieve the nurse of the responsibility for this intravenous therapy.

Factors that influence intravenous flow rate include positional changes, change in needle position, constricting tape, height of the solution bottle, a nonpatent air vent, and a nonpatent needle. Local infiltration of fluids into the subcutaneous tissue, inflammation of the vein (phlebitis), air embolus, and circulatory overload are potential complications of intravenous therapy.

Clients receiving intravenous therapy should be told of realistic expectations of pain, encouraged to exercise areas which will not dislodge the needle, and assessed every hour for any complications.

Intravenous therapy is a temporary means of sustenance and can replace fluids, electrolytes, glucose, and some vitamins but not protein and fat. **Total parenteral nutrition** (TPN) can supply total nutritional requirements. Intravenous therapy is also an efficient route for medication administration. Medicine may be added to the solution chamber, to a volume control chamber, a medication pump, piggyback technique, or directly into the venipuncture sight (bolus or heparin lock technique). There are very specific techniques for administering medication intravenously, and the nurse must be aware that medication actions and adverse effects will occur quickly.

A particular form of intravenous therapy is the **blood transfusion.** Blood transfusions consist of either whole blood (plasma, blood cells, and all other blood constituents), packed red blood cells (concentration of red blood cells after the plasma has been removed), washed packed red blood cells (antibodies have been removed to prevent allergic reactions), white blood cells (leukocytes only), plasma (blood cells removed), cryoprecipitate (contains specific clotting factors, and platelets.

Administering blood requires two people (doctors or nurses) to check that the blood received from the blood bank has been properly cross-matched with the recipient's blood. The baseline temperature and the pulse and blood pressure values are established for comparison during the transfusion. Blood is administered using a special transfusion set with a blood filter and Y-type tubing so that normal saline can be infused before and after the blood.

In order to prevent *incompatible blood reactions* (hemolytic reaction), the person who is to receive a blood transfusion must first have a sample of blood drawn; this blood is examined to determine the type **(blood type)** and then is mixed with the donor blood and observed for a hemolytic reaction **(cross matching).** Allergic reactions and pyrogenic reactions may also occur. In any of these events the transfusion should be immediately discontinued, and the physician notified. Further complications of blood transfusions include circulatory overload, excess of potassium, calcium citrate reactions, and hemosiderosis.

Today, blood donors are carefully screened before donating their blood, and the blood is further screened for syphilis, hepatitis, and AIDS after it has been collected.

Shock (inadequate circulation to the body cells) may be due to blood loss, fluid loss, cardiac failure, neurogenic shock, septic shock, or obstructive shock. In early shock the body tries to **compensate** using generalized **vasoconstriction.** However, continued fluid loss will result in death. Symptoms of shock are decreasing blood pressure, increasing pulse rate, a decreasing pulse pressure, decreasing urine output, restlessness, and anxiety. Nursing interventions for the client in shock include administering oxygen via face mask, promoting the supine position, administering intravenous fluids (possibly blood transfusions), and providing adequate (not extreme) warmth.

DRILL AND PRACTICE QUESTIONS FOR REVIEW

Complete the statements below.

1. The two major fluid compartments in the body are the _____ compartment and the _____ compartment.

2. The term used to refer to the body's ability to maintain balance despite disturbances is _____.

3. _____ water loss is water lost from sweat and the lungs.

4. Sodium and potassium are _____, while chlorides and phosphates are _____.

5. An electrolyte which is influential in the health of bone and teeth is _____.

6. A client who is experiencing an increased urine output and subsequent fluid loss is said to be _____.

7. Excessive drinking of large amounts of fluids because of thirst is called _____.

8. The three buffer systems in the body which regulate acid-base balance are the _____, _____, and _____.

9. Dorsiflexing the foot as an assessment for calcium deficits is called the test for _____.

10. _____ is excess fluid in the interstitial spaces.

11. _____ is an accumulation of fluid in the abdominal cavity.

12. Two foods high in potassium are _____ and _____.

13. Infants with electrolyte imbalances may be given a solution called _____.

14. The three most common sites for an intravenous infusion are the _____, _____, and _____.

15. Another name for a scalp vein needle is a _____ needle.

16. An intravenous solution of 10 percent dextrose in water is hypertonic, and an intravenous solution of 5 percent dextrose in water is _____.

17. The total intravenous fluid volume to be infused is 1000 ml. in the next ten hours. the drop factor is 10 gtts. per ml. Therefore, you would regulate the intravenous to infuse at _____ gtts, per minute.

18. An accumulation of intravenous solution in the subcutaneous tissue is referred to as an _____.

19. If your client has signs of a phlebitis at the intravenous site, you should _____ the infusion and _____ the needle.

20. In order to determine if a recipient's blood is compatible with a donor's blood a _____ and _____ is done.

21. For adults receiving a blood transfusion, a No. _____ needle is used; and for infants, a No. _____ is used.

22. A blood transfusion should be completed within _____ hours' time.

23. If your client who is having a blood transfusion develops hives and itching, this condition is probably a (an) _____ reaction.

24. Shock which is caused by dilation of the peripheral circulation is called _____ shock.

25. The best position for the person in shock is the _____ position.

Determine whether the following statements are TRUE or FALSE.

1. Women's bodies contain proportionally less water than men's bodies.

2. An increased production of ADH (antidiuretic hormone) will cause fluid loss.

3. An increased production of aldosterone causes the body to secrete sodium and water and to retain potassium.

4. The normal pH of the blood is 7.35 to 7.45.

5. Excessive use of diuretics may lead to dehydration.

6. Diarrhea may lead to fluid losses but not electrolyte losses.

7. With an increased fluid volume, the pulse is often bounding.

8. A dehydrated client will have poor skin turgor, dry skin, dry lips, and in extreme cases, sunken eyeballs.

9. Diarrhea may be fatal in the infant.

10. Excessive vomiting may lead to metabolic alkalosis.

11. Generalized edema is referred to as anasarca.

12. To reduce the fluid load in the body, a salt-restricted diet may be prescribed.

13. Daily weight measurements are a better indicator of fluid loss or fluid gain than is an intake and output record.

14. Intravenous potassium must be given very carefully because excess amounts of potassium can cause cardiac arrhythmias.

15. Intracath needles are thought to infiltrate less often than metal needles because of their ability to bend.

16. Intravenous therapy can supply a person with all the fluids and nutrients necessary to sustain life.

17. Nurses need to wear gloves during venipuncture only when they are administering blood products.

18. Before venipuncture, the skin is cleansed with either 70 percent alcohol or povidone iodine solution.

19. Ringer's solution is a hypertonic intravenous solution.

20. Filters on intravenous tubings are designed to remove any bacteria inadvertently left in the solution after sterilization.

21. Commonly, the rate of a KVO infusion is set at 40 to 50 ml. per hour.

22. When administering plasma, the nurse should follow standards for administering intravenous solutions, not for administering blood products.

23. The intravenous tubing used for blood transfusions should be primed first with 5 percent dextrose in water.

24. An increasing pulse rate and a decreasing blood pressure are indicators of shock.

25. The client in shock should be given supplemental oxygen.

Situations

Situation 1

Mr. Meyer has been admitted to the hospital because of kidney failure. For the next few days he will be undergoing several diagnostic tests in order to determine the appropriate treatment course. In the meanwhile his physician has ordered that Mr. Meyer's daily fluid intake be restricted to 900 ml. List all pertinent nursing considerations specific to this fluid restriction.

Situation 2

Mrs. Brown is complaining of pain in her antecubital space where her intravenous is infusing. The nurse examines her arm and notices redness and swelling around the needle insertion site and decides to remove the needle from this site. In the appropriate order, list the steps the nurse should take to remove an intravenous needle.

ANSWERS TO DRILL AND PRACTICE QUESTIONS

Completion Exercises

1. extracellular, intracellular
2. homeostasis
3. Insensible
4. cation, anin
5. calcium
6. diuresing
7. polydipsia
8. buffer salts, kidney, respirations
9. clonus
10. Edema
11. Ascites
12. bananas, orange juice
13. Pediolyte
14. hand, forearm, antecubital space
15. butterfly
16. isotonic
17. 16 or 17
18. infiltration
19. discontinue, remove
20. blood typing, cross matching
21. 18, 20
22. four

23. allergic

24. neurogenic

25. supine

True/False Exercises

1.	T	13.	T
2.	F	14.	T
3.	F	15.	T
4.	T	16.	F
5.	T	17.	F
6.	F	18.	T
7.	T	19.	F
8.	T	20.	F
9.	T	21.	F
10.	F	22.	F
11.	T	23.	F
12.	T	24.	T
		25.	T

Situations

Situation 1

- explain the fluid restriction regime to Mr. Meyer
- explain the fluid restrictions to Mr. Meyer's family and ask for their cooperation and encouragement
- determine if Mr. Meyer would prefer to be given his fluids spaced throughout the day or to have fluids less frequently in larger amounts
- be sure Mr. Meyer is not given foods that will increase his thirst, such as dairy products and those high in salt and sugar
- keep water pitchers and other beverages out of sight
- ask the dietary department not to park the service cart and its aromas of coffee near Mr. Meyer's room
- offer mouthwashes often and remind Mr. Meyer not to swallow
- do not offer Mr. Meyer ice chips because they will add up to significant amounts of water

Situation 2

1. Tell Mrs. Brown what you are about to do.
2. Put on gloves.
3. Clamp off the tubing.
4. Remove the dressing and the tape.
5. Press an alcohol compress against the puncture site.
6. Pull the needle out and back against the surface of the skin.
7. Apply pressure to the site until any bleeding stops.
8. In the meantime, check the needle to make sure it is intact.
9. Apply a bandaid to the puncture site if Mrs. Brown wishes

Chapter 43

CARDIOVASCULAR FUNCTION

MAJOR NURSING CONCEPTS

Cardiovascular functioning is necessary for life and depends on a functioning heart, blood vessels, and blood. **Cardiac output** is the amount of blood pumped from the left ventricle of the heart times the heart rate per minute.

Cardiovascular assessment begins with a health history and should include asking about unusual fatigue, squatting in children, "skipped beats," cold, tingling, or numbness of the extremities, vertigo (dizziness), and stress. The physical examination should encompass heart rate and quality, blood pressure, buccal membrane and skin color (paleness, cyanosis), capillary filling, **clubbing of fingers,** diminished hair growth on legs, urine output, and edema. **Pitting edema** refers to an edema so intense that when your finger is pressed against the skin, an indentation remains. Edema is rated on a four point scale; 4+ is the greatest degree of edema, and 0 means no edema.

A nurse's cardiovascular assessment should also include the presence or absence of varicosities. **Varicose veins** are tortuous, distended veins. Clients with varicosities complain of aching legs and are at greater risk of developing blood clots because of sluggish blood flow through these damaged veins. **Arteriosclerosis** (hardening of the arteries) and **atherosclerosis** (fatty plaque deposits in the arteries) decrease circulation to the major organs and can sometimes be assessed by the nurse using the capillary refill technique.

Venous pressure is measured in centimeters of water by a CVP (**central venous pressure**) catheter placed in the superior or inferior vena cava. **Pulmonary artery pressure** can be measured in a similar manner as the central venous pressure, except this necessitates using a Swan-Ganz catheter which has been threaded into the pulmonary artery. Both the CVP and the pulmonary artery pressure give the nurse information about how well the heart is able to handle the circulating fluid load.

Nursing diagnoses pertinent to cardiovascular malfunctioning include "alteration in cardiac output" and "alteration in tissue perfusion."

Nursing interventions specific to cardiovascular function are often age-related.

Cardiac anomalies are a common type of **birth** defect. While most can be corrected with surgery, nurses need to understand that this diagnosis is extremely frightening to parents and nurses must be ready to offer a great deal of nursing support. **Children** may develop damage to their heart valves as a complication of a streptococci (beta hemolytic A) infection of the ears or throat. Nurses should teach and encourage parents to have their children seen by a physician for ear and throat pains. Hypertension may develop during childhood, and it is often, but not always, related to obesity and excess sodium intake. Nurses need to counsel parents and children on the importance of low fat and moderate salt intake in their diets.

Hypertension and myocardial infarction are major cardiovascular health problems seen in **adults.** Nurses often need to teach clients with hypertension the importance of continuing with their medication regime as well as devising strategies designed to remind the client to take his medicine each day. Clients who have experienced a myocardial infarction are helped by nurses to live a full life within the limits of their cardiovascular function. Nursing care for the **older adult** may include rehabilitation measures after a stroke.

Other nursing interventions include **antiembolic stockings** and ace bandages to promote venous circulation. Be sure these stockings and bandages fit properly and are applied smoothly while the client is in the supine position. **Fowler's positions** reduce the workload of the heart and should be encouraged when not contraindicated. Circulation to all areas of the body can be checked by the capillary refill technique, palpating for warmth, and asking clients if they feel tingling or numbness. Elevating a body part decreases the edema present. Muscle contractions during exercise (passive and active range-of-motion, wiggling toes) improve venous circulation and should be encouraged when medically permitted.

Nursing interventions for the client who is experiencing blood loss include supporting the supine position, intravenous therapy, various medications, and direct pressure to the bleeding site. **Nosebleeds** may be treated by high Fowler's position, pressure to the sides of the nose, cold compresses, and attendance by the nurse to decrease anxiety.

Phlebitis (inflammation of a vein) and **thrombophlebitis** (inflammation of a vein with an accompanying blood clot) are best prevented using such methods as range-of-motion exercises, antiembolic stockings, and changing intravenous sites every seventy-two hours. The presence of thrombophlebitis in a leg vein can be assessed using the **Homans' sign.**

DRILL AND PRACTICE QUESTIONS FOR REVIEW

Complete the statements below.

1. Spoon-shaped fingertips are often referred to as _____ fingers.

2. _____ is a type of vertigo caused by a dropping blood pressure on arising.

3. A person who has a compelling sense of time and a great need to succeed is a Type _____ personality, according to Friedman and Roseman.

4. Extensive edema in which a pressed finger to the skin leaves an indentation mark is called _____ edema.

5. The normal central venous pressure should be between _____ and _____ centimeters of water.

6. A hemolytic streptococcal infection which affects the heart valves is _____.

7. A body position which decreases the work load of the heart is the _____.

8. Antiembolic stockings should be removed at least _____ times a day in order to assess the underlying skin.

9. During the application of ace bandages to the legs, the client should be in the _____ position.

10. In order to promote vasoconstriction, the nurse may utilize the application of _____.

11. Clients who are bleeding from their nose should be placed in the _____ position.

12. Signs of phlebitis include _____, _____, and _____ in the area.

Determine whether the following statements are TRUE or FALSE

1. Vasodilation of an area causes warmth and redness to that area.

2. In an ambulatory client, edema is most likely to develop in the feet and lower legs.

3. A decrease in cardiac output will result in an increase in urinary output.

4. Nurses should encourage clients with varicosities of the lower legs to avoid standing in one place for long periods of time.

5. The intravenous flow on a central venous pressure line should infuse into the client only when pressure readings are being performed.

6. Hypertension never develops in children.

7. Clients with decreased cardiac function should be encouraged to assume the supine position.

8. In an effort to decrease the amount of edema, the nurse may elevate the edematous body part.

9. The most effective way to halt bleeding is to apply a tourniquet proximal to the bleeding site.

10. Thrombophlebitis is a serious problem because the blood clot may travel to other areas of the body such as the lungs, heart, or brain.

11. Nursing interventions for the client with phlebitis of the leg include gentle massage to the leg.

12. Bedrest increases one's risk for developing thrombophlebitis.

Situations

Situation 1

Mrs. Mason is a sixty-six-year-old housewife who has been on bedrest for the past three days because she has had a myocardial infarction. While caring for Mrs. Moore today, the nurse noted a positive Homans' sign in Mrs. Moore's left leg. Develop a nursing care plan for Mrs. Moore specific to this development of phlebitis.

Situation 2

Mr. Richards is admitted to the intensive care unit because of significant blood loss from a gastric ulcer. In order to assess carefully how well his heart is handling the large number of intravenous fluids that he is being given, a central venous pressure line was inserted. Describe the steps the nurse would take while taking a central venous pressure reading.

ANSWERS TO DRILL AND PRACTICE QUESTIONS

Completion Exercises

1. clubbed
2. Orthostatic hypotension
3. "A"
4. pitting
5. five, fifteen
6. rheumatic fever
7. Fowler's
8. two
9. supine
10. cold
11. high-Fowler's
12. warmth, pain, redness

True/False Exercises

1.	T	7.	F
2.	T	8.	T
3.	F	9.	F
4.	T	10.	T
5.	F	11.	F
6.	F	12.	T

Situations

Situation 1

Nursing Assessments:

Assess left leg for redness, swelling, and warmth.

Ask Mrs. Moore if she has pain in her left leg

Check Homans' signs in both legs every eight hours.

Assess respiratory rate, level of consciousness, and presence of chest pain to determine whether any complications of thrombophlebitis have occurred (blood clot to lungs, heart, or brain).

Nursing Diagnosis:

Potential for injury (blood clot to vital organ—heart attack, stroke, etc.).

Nursing Goals:

Client will not develop complications.

Client will not develop phlebitis in her other leg.

Client's Homans' signs will return to normal within five days.

Nursing Interventions

    Continued assessments (as above) for phlebitis.

    Bedrest and immobilization of the left leg.

    Application of heat to the left leg.

    Be prepared to administer anticoagulants as prescribed by the physician.

    Range-of-motion exercises to the right leg.

Situation 2

- ascertain that the zero mark on the manometer is at the same level as the atria of Mr. Richards' heart (midaxillary line at the third or fourth interspace)
- turn the stopcock so that the intravenous fluid flows into the manometer
- fill the manometer to the 30 centimeter level
- turn the stopcock to open the flow into the patient
- watch the fluid as it falls, and note at what number of the manometer the fluid level rests (this is Mr. Richards' CVP0)
- be aware that slight fluctuations in the fluid level are due to normal respirations
- reverse the stopcock to reopen the fluid between the intravenous fluid and the catheter

Chapter 44

HEAT AND COLD THERAPY

MAJOR NURSING CONCEPTS

Heat and cold applications are used to reduce pain and inflammation, and to facilitate healing. It is important for nurses to understand the purposes and implications of heat and cold applications in order to plan appropriate safe care.

Thermal regulation and nursing implications across the life span are as follows:

- The infant should never be left alone with any source of heat or cold.

- The toddler/preschooler should never play games with electrical sources of heat application. Wall plugs should be used to cover outlets.

- The school-ager/adolescent may consider application of heat or cold unnecessary. They may need play activities during treatment.

- The adult needs to be encouraged to accept heat and cold applications as therapy and may need diversional therapy during treatment.

- The older adult may have decreased skin sensation to applications of heat and cold.

Assessment for the application of heat and cold includes skin appearance prior to application and approximately ten minutes after application, for color, temperature, integrity, and sensation.

Effects of heat application include the promotion of healing, muscle relaxation, pain relief, vasodilation of peripheral arterioles, increased blood flow, increased cell metabolism, and increased need for oxygen by the cells. Heat application should be no hotter than 43.3 degrees C (110 degrees F). Extreme heat may cause burns and interfere with circulation. Heat reaches its maximum effect in approximately twenty to thirty minutes. After approximately one hour vasoconstriction (secondary effect) occurs, depriving affected areas of oxygen and nutrition.

There are two types of heat application.

- **Moist heat** can be applied by soaks, compresses, and baths (sitz, whirlpool). Moist heat penetrates deeper than dry heat; it transfers heat to body by conduction. There is less body fluid loss and less sweating, and it is easier to apply.

- **Dry heat** can be applied by heat lamp, heating pads, heat cradles, diathermy, ultraviolet light, and hot water bags. Dry heat may cause burns and increased fluid loss due to evaporation of perspiration at site of application. It does not penetrate as deep as moist heat, so that it may not be as effective in relieving deep muscle pain. There is danger of electrical shock when using equipment requiring electricity.

Effects of cold application include decreases of blood flow and cell perfusion, reduction of pain and prevention of edema. Application of cold reaches maximum effect in thirty to sixty minutes. After approximately one hour, vasodilation (secondary effect) occurs. Applying ice directly to skin can cause frostbite or skin cell destruction.

There are two types of cold application.

- **Moist cold** can be applied by baths or compresses; it may cause burns.
- **Dry cold** can be applied by ice bags or chemical packs.

Before applying heat or cold, the following factors should be assessed:

- individual temperature tolerance
- circulating adaptation capacity
- neurological response capability
- decreased pain sensation due to medication
- age
- presence of healing tissue
- presence of malignancy (cancer)
- kidney function
- edema
- pain

Nurses should be aware of principles of safety that are the basis for safe, comfortable heat and cold application.

- Avoid use of metal safety pins to anchor electrical wiring for heating pads.
- When using a heat lamp, remain with the client to prevent burns.
- Ice packs should be covered with a towel to prevent skin cell destruction.
- Apply heat or cold for twenty minutes to avoid secondary reactions.
- Be wary of clients on analgesics, sedatives, or hypnotics, because they may have altered perceptions of heat or cold.
- Do not use electrical equipment near water.

DRILL AND PRACTICE QUESTIONS FOR REVIEW

Completion Questions

1. Older adults may have a _____ sensation for heat or cold.
2. During the application of heat or cold, assess the client for _____.
3. Local application of heat causes _____, _____, and _____.
4. Heat reaches its maximum effect in _____ to _____ minutes.
5. After prolonged heat application, the secondary effect of _____ occurs.
6. Extreme heat causes _____.

7. Heat facilitates wound healing by _____.

8. Local application of cold causes _____.

9. Cold applications are used to _____ and _____.

10. Three factors that should be assessed before applying heat or cold are _____, _____, and _____.

11. Heat may be applied as _____ or _____ heat.

12. To prevent cooling of warm compresses, cover the outside with a _____ pad.

13. The temperature in a whirlpool bath should not exceed _____.

14. Paraffin baths are effective in _____ and _____.

15. Three examples of dry heat are _____, _____, and _____.

16. Hot-water bags should be used cautiously because _____.

17. Diathermy is _____.

True/False Questions

1. Human skin contains about three times as many receptors for heat as it does for cold.

2. Extreme changes in heat or cold stimulate pain receptors.

3. Infants may be left alone while receiving heat lamp therapy because they cannot fall out of their crib.

4. Prolonged applications of heat increases oxygen and nutrition to the area.

5. Applications of cold reach their maximum effect in thirty to sixty minutes.

6. People with arteriosclerosis have increased blood supply to body parts.

7. Ice may be applied directly to the skin to prevent swelling.

8. Infants and older adults may have a decreased ability to perceive pain from heat or cold.

9. Heat should be used cautiously with a malignancy.

10. Heat application can cause changes in the filtering function of the kidneys.

11. Heat should be routinely applied to the abdomen when clients complain of pain.

12. Applications of heat and cold are usually ordered five times a day.

13. Wet heat penetrates deeper than dry heat.

14. Clients with cardiac pacemakers should not receive diathermy treatment.

15. When applying cold to a large body surface, apply a colder compress to the forehead.

Situation

Gene Grown is a thirty-five-year-old patient hospitalized for external hemorrhoids (distended tortuous veins located distal to the anal sphincter). He complains of perianal pain and itching. The physician has prescribed warm sitz baths for twenty minutes three times a day. As the nurse caring for Mr. Brown, describe the procedure for warm sitz baths and include the rationale for each step.

ANSWERS TO DRILL AND PRACTICE QUESTIONS

Completion Exercises

1. deceased
2. circulatory change; change in skin temperature, color, and integrity
3. vasodilation, increased cell metabolism, and increased cell need for oxygen
4. twenty to thirty minutes
5. vasoconstriction
6. vasoconstriction
7. drawing lymph, leukocytes, and antibodies to the area
8. vasoconstriction
9. reduce pain and swelling
10. temperature tolerance, circulation, age, and presence of malignancy
11. moist or dry
12. waterproof
13. 100 degrees F
14. relieving pain and increasing mobility
15. heat lamps, cradles, and heating pads
16. they are not temperature controlled
17. a change of electrical energy into heat energy

True/False Exercises

1.	F	8.	T
2.	T	9.	T
3.	F	10.	T
4.	F	11.	F
5.	T	12.	F
6.	F	13.	T
7.	F	14.	T
		15.	T

Situation

1. Wash hands, identify the patient, and explain the procedure. This procedure is done to ensure patient safety, facilitate compliance, and reduce anxiety.
2. Fill the basin with warm water, no higher than 110 degrees F. Extreme heat can interfere with circulation and cause serious burns.
3. Provide privacy in order to maintain the patient's self-esteem.
4. Cover the patient with a bath blanket and assist to a comfortable position in the sitz bath; pad any pressure areas.
5. Stay with Mr.. Brown during entire procedure and observe him for signs of weakness, dizziness, or lightheadedness. Changes in circulatory level have a sedative effect and may produce fainting.

6. Carefully maintain temperature of the water.
7. Assist Mr. Brown out of the sitz bath into a dry gown and back to bed. Instruct him to remain in bed until normal circulation returns and any feelings of weakness or dizziness have disappeared.

Chapter 45

OXYGEN AND CARBON DIOXIDE REGUALTION

NOTE TO STUDENT

Be sure to review the anatomy and physiology of the respiratory system before beginning this chapter. Review suctioning procedures 45-1, 45-2, and 45-3 because these procedures are often life-saving, but they are not without complications.

MAJOR NURSING CONCEPTS

Assessing respiratory function and maintaining oxygenation are always **priority nursing considerations.**

The **health history** should contain questions about smoking, occupation, and the number of pillows the client uses for sleep. Shortness of breath, fatigue, orthopnea (difficulty breathing in a supine position), and chronic cough are symptoms which may indicate serious respiratory disease. Parents of infants should be questioned about difficulty in feeding, since a baby cannot suck easily if he or she is experiencing any respiratory distress. Frequent upper respiratory tract diseases may indicate allergy, exposure to a polluted environment, or decreased immunosuppressive activity.

The nurse's **physical examination** pertinent to respiratory function encompasses several factors. A client in respiratory difficulty may display signs such as restlessness, an anxious expression, dyspnea, nasal flaring, and an inability to exercise. Inspect the chest contour for lack of symmetry, uneven chest expansion, presence of a **"barrel"** chest (increased anteroposterior diameter), and **pectus excavatum** (decreased anterioposterior diameter). Look for **retraction** (supracostal, subcostal, intracostal). Observe for cyanosis (bluish discoloration of skin, nailbeds, or buccal membranes), "clubbing" of the fingertips, and breath odor (alcohol, sweet smell of metabolic acidosis). Noting a client's speech pattern such as the inability to complete a sentence without pausing for breath and the strength and pitch of the voice is important. Palpation for **fremitus** (vibrations felt by placing the palms of your hands on the client's chest) increases when fluid is present in the chest. Auscultating the sounds of respiration by using a stethoscope is an important nursing assessment because abnormal sounds are often serious. Any **cough** should be assessed for production of mucous, hemoptysis, characteristic patterns (croup or whooping cough), and predisposing factors such as cigarette smoke or position.

Pulmonary function studies determine one's breathing capacity using spirometers. **Arterial blood gas** reports give you information about how well the lungs are able to transfer oxygen (normal PaO_2 = 80 to 100) to the blood and remove carbon dioxide (normal $PaCO_2$ = 38 to 42) from the blood. Falling PaO_2 levels and rising $PaCO_2$ levels often indicate respiratory malfunction. The lungs play an important role in regulating acid-base balance by regulating carbon dioxide elimination. Hyperventilation promotes the elimination of CO_2 (CO_2 is necessary for the production of acid) and leads to alkalosis, while hypoventilation promotes the retention of CO_2 and leads to acidosis.

221

Nursing diagnoses relevant to oxygen and carbon dioxide regulation are "ineffective airway clearance," "ineffective breathing patterns," and "impaired gas exchange."

Oxygen and carbon dioxide regulation in the **fetus** is dependent on the placenta-uterine interface. Any condition or situation which causes the mother's oxygen level to decrease will have serious consequences for the fetus. A **newborn's** respiratory rate is fast (thirty to fifty breaths per minutes) and may be slightly irregular. Since **infants** are nose breathers, their nasal passages must be kept clean and open whenever they develop a "cold." Upper respiratory infections may lead to feeding problems and cause excoriation to the skin under the nose and lead to otitis media. **Toddlers** and **preschoolers** are often exposed to and develop upper respiratory infections which, if accompanied by a sore throat, may indicate a streptococcal infection requiring antibiotic therapy. **School-agers** and **adolescents** continue to have upper respiratory infections and need to be taught the dangers of smoking, since some develop asthma during these years. Fractured ribs and pneumonia in the **young adult** cause respiratory distress. The **middle-aged** smokers are prone to lung cancer and emphysema (overdistention of the alveoli). The **older adult** develops diminished respiratory function because of inactivity, diminished rib cage expansion, and arteriosclerosis.

Clients who have difficulty breathing are naturally **fearful.** Provide a stress-free environment and attend the person frequently. Provide frequent mouth care to prevent mucosal cracks and odor. **Adequate hydration** keeps respiratory secretions (sputum) moist and therefore readily movable.

Expectoration of secretions from the respiratory tract is important in order to keep the airways clear. Deep breathing and coughing (use the **"splinting"** technique for postoperative clients), turning immobilized clients every two hours, and encouraging and assisting with ambulation promote the mobilization and **expectoration** of secretions.

Aerosol therapy via **nebulizers** provides a stream of moistened air into the respiratory tract which loosens secretions and may deliver antibiotic therapy to the lungs. A **humidifier** delivers moisture to the room air and is a less efficient method of liquifying secretions and administering medications. **Intermittent Positive Pressure Breathing** (IPPB) machines deliver oxygen, humidification, and medication to the respiratory tract under pressure. Nurses should observe for signs of complications from nebulizers, IPPB machines, and humidifiers, such as infections, overload of fluid to the lungs, bronchial irritation, or systemic effects of the added medications.

Postural drainage uses gravity, via different body positions, to mobilize secretions in the respiratory tract. **Clapping, vibration,** and **percussion** may be used with or without postural drainage. Oral and nasal suctioning using a bulb syringe is very gentle and frequently used with infants. **Suctioning** (oral, nasal, endotracheal) removes secretions from the respiratory tract using a catheter and suction machine. These suctioning procedures, which are used when the respiratory tract is obstructed with secretions, require good technique and expose the client to risks such as trauma to the airway, hypoxemia (lowered oxygen in the blood), alveolar collapse, vagal stimulation (may result in serious bradycardia), hypotension (from severe bradycardia), and paroxysmal cough (spasm like coughing).

Additional **nursing interventions** for improving aeration of the lungs include **incentive spirometers** (colorful plastic devices which encourage people to inhale deeply), promoting a mid to high **Fowler's position,** administering analgesic medications to clients when pain is interfering with good respiratory function, and **breathing techniques** such as abdominal muscle breathing and "pursed lip" breathing.

The **administration of oxygen** will improve a client's respiratory function unless conditions in which diffusion across the alveoli is the basic problem. Blood gas levels should be used to determine the necessity and the effectiveness of oxygen therapy. Oxygen therapy may cause respiratory arrest in clients with chronic obstructive lung disease, blindness from **retrolental fibroplasia** in premature infants, **oxygen toxicity** with long-term high concentration use, and atelectasis.

Physicians may prescribe one of several methods for oxygen administration such as nasal prongs, nasopharyngeal catheters, oxygen masks, oxygen tents, oxygen hoods, Venturi masks, and nonrebreathing masks and rebreathing masks. Mist tents provide moisture without oxygen. Ventilators deliver oxygen under pressure. Excessive pressure from a ventilator may collapse a lung. **Safety considerations** during oxygen administration include labeled and well-ventilated rooms, no smoking, no incense, no candle burning, grounded electrical plugs on all equipment, and the use of only cotton blankets.

An **obstructed airway** may be due to an accumulation of respiratory secretions, aspiration of fluids, food, or a foreign object; it is always an emergency situation. In order to dislodge a completely obstructed airway, use the **Heimlich maneuver** except for infants, with whom it is more effective to turn the baby head down and administer back blows.

During **cardiopulmonary arrest** the nurse should first open the person's airway (hyperextend the neck or bring the lower jaw forward) and then begin mouth-to-mouth resuscitation (using a one-way mask or an Ambu bag). Next, provide circulation using cardiac compressions between respirations. The next step in cardiopulmonary resuscitation will be the administration of medications, usually via an intravenous line.

Care of a client with a **tracheotomy** (permanent incision into the trachea) or a tracheostomy (temporary incision into the anterior trachea) includes sterile suctioning of excess respiratory secretions, attending the client frequently to decrease fears, teaching the client to talk by placing his finger over the tracheostomy opening, cleaning the tube, and changing dressings prn.

DRILL AND PRACTICE QUESTIONS FOR REVIEW

Complete the statements below.

1. The _____ bronchus is straighter and wider than the other bronchus.

2. Infants usually breathe through their _____.

3. When the subcostal, supracostal, or intracostal spaces are sucked in during respiration, this procedure is called _____.

4. _____ is difficulty breathing except in an upright position.

5. _____ is the cessation of breathing.

6. The normal PaO2 is _____ to _____.

7. When the body is depleted of hydrogen ions, a state of _____ exists.

8. A lipoprotein produced by the fetus at about thirty-five weeks of age that helps to prevent alveoli from closing is _____.

9. _____ is an exercise often suggested for people with lung illnesses.

10. _____ is the term used when raising mucus from the respiratory tract.

11. When assisting a postoperative client to cough and deep breathe, it is useful to _____ the incisional area to decrease any pain.

12. A method used to deliver miniscule droplets into the respiratory tract is called _____.

13. It is safer to use _____ water in a humidifier.

14. A mucus mobilization technique using the principle of gravity is called _____.

15. Trauma to the airways during suctioning can be reduced by first _____ the catheter.

16. When handling nasal oxygen equipment, the nurse should wear _____.

17. The oxygen administration method useful for the hyperventilating clients is _____.

18. The highest concentration of oxygen that can be achieved in a tent is _____ percent.

19. One way to determine whether a person has a completely obstructed airway is to ask the person to _____.

20. A tube that is inserted via the mouth into the trachea for purposes of keeping the upper airways open is called a (an) _____.

Determine if the following statements are TRUE or FALSE.

1. Difficulty with the diffusion of gases across the alveoli membrane increases in the presence of secretions.

2. Marijuana cigarettes do not cause damage to the respiratory tract.

3. Infants normally use their abdominal muscles to assist in breathing.

4. Cyanosis is a late sign of oxygen lack.

5. Breath sounds are absent when the lung is collapsed.

6. The normal PaC02 is 80 to 100.

7. Hypoventilation often predisposes a person to acidosis.

8. The normal respiratory rate for newborns is twenty to thirty respirations per minute.

9. In order to prevent skin excoriation under the nose of a newborn with a cold, the nurse should instruct the mother to apply Vaseline to the area.

10. Children with chronic lung disease should be encouraged to participate in extracurricular activities.

11. All respiratory distress brings with it some psychological distress.

12. Handwashing is necessary to prevent contamination from clients expectorating sputum even when they use tissues.

13. Administration of aerosol medication caries the same nursing responsibility as does administration of other forms of medications.

14. Tap water is used in nebulizers and humidifiers in health-care agencies.

15. Gurgling respirations, increased tactile fremitus, and rhonchi are indications that the client may need suctioning.

16. In order to reduce the risk of hypoxemia, the nurse can administer oxygen before and after suctioning.

17. Incentive spirometers promote full respiratory expiration.

18. Oxygen administered via a Venturi mask need not be humidified.

19. Clients should be encouraged to wear wool blankets and sweaters to provide warmth when in an oxygen tent.

20. If two people certified in cardiopulmonary resuscitation are present, the first rescuer can ventilate at the same time as the second rescuer is doing cardiac compression.

Situations

Situation 1

Miss Shanley is a forty-three-year-old school teacher who went to the emergency room complaining of a nagging cough, fever, and fatigue. After a chest X-ray, it was determined that Miss Shanley had pneumonia and she was to be admitted to the hospital for antibiotic therapy. Describe your nursing care plan, specifically addressing oxygen and carbon dioxide regulation, for Miss Shanley.

Situation 2

Mr. McNulty has been admitted to the coronary care unit with a myocardial infarction (heart attack). His physician has ordered 6 liters of nasal oxygen to be administered via a nasopharyngeal catheter. List the steps the nurse should take when administering oxygen via a nasopharyngeal catheter.

ANSWERS TO DRILL AND PRACTICE QUESTIONS

Completion Exercises

1. right
2. noses
3. retraction
4. Orthopnea
5. Apnea
6. 80, 100
7. alkalosis
8. surfactant
9. Swimming
10. Expectorating
11. splint
12. ultrasonic nebulization
13. cold
14. postural drainage
15. lubricating
16. gloves
17. rebreathing bag
18. 50

19. speak

20. endotracheal tube

True/False Exercises

1. T	11. T
2. F	12. T
3. T	13. T
4. T	14. F
5. T	15. T
6. F	16. T
7. T	17. F
8. F	18. T
9. F	19. F
10. T	20. F

Situations

Situation 1

Nursing Assessments:
- assess respiratory rate
- assess skin, lips, nailbeds, and buccal mucosa for cyanosis
- assess for tactile fremitus
- auscultate breath sounds for rales or rhonchi
- assess production of sputum
- assess color, odor, and amount of sputum
- check doctor's orders to determine if sputum for culture and sensitivity is needed
- assess blood gas reports

Nursing Diagnoses:
- ineffective breathing pattern (dyspnea)
- impaired gas exchange

Nursing Interventions:
- assist with Fowler's position
- encourage fluids to liquify secretions
- offer frequent oral hygiene
- use percussion, cupping, and vibration to loosen secretions
- encourage Miss Shanley to expectorate sputum, and give her tissues and a paper disposal bag
- to decrease pain, splint Miss Shanley's chest with pillows when she coughs
- attend Miss Shanley frequently in order to decrease any anxiety associated with respiratory difficulty
- medicate with antibiotics and expectorants according to her physician's orders

Situation 2

1. Inform Mr. McNulty what you are about to do.
2. Measure the proper distance between the nose and the earlobe.
3. Coat the catheter lightly with a water-soluble lubricant.
4. Tell Mr. McNulty that passage of the catheter will cause a temporary discomfort such as tickling.

5. Put on a pair of gloves.
6. Gently insert the catheter.
7. Bring the catheter to the side of Mr. McNulty's nose and tape it to his cheek.
8. Adjust oxygen flow to 6 liters per minute.
9. Replace the catheter with a fresh one in the other nostril every eight hours.

Chapter 46

GASTROINTESTINAL ELIMINATION

MAJOR NURSING CONCEPTS

Norman **defecation** involves the expulsion of waste products (soft **feces** or stool) from the intestinal tract (number of bowel movements varies from person to person). Defecation depends on the presence of **peristalsis** (waves of intestinal contraction and relaxation), normal sensory nerves, and sphincter control. Peristalsis is facilitated by activity, and its presence is determined with auscultation of bowel sounds and/or passage of flatus. Defecation occurs more easily with the use of the sitting position, uninjured and nontender abdominal muscles, and the presence of soft stool (facilitated by having adequate fiber—fruits and vegetables are good sources—and water in the diet). **Straining** to pass stool (e.g., when stools are hard) can precipitate a **Valsalva maneuver** (breathing out against a closed glottis), which can cause an increase in intrathoracic pressure, and a subsequent decrease in cardiac output and fainting. Exhaling through the mouth when straining can help prevent the Valsalva response.

The first stool passed by a **newborn** is called **meconium** (normally black, odorless, and passed within twenty-four hours of birth). Stools progress from loose green stools to loose yellow stools (about six per day). **Infants** appear to strain with passage of stool, but this action is normal. **Diarrhea** (more frequent, acidic, loose stools) can quickly cause skin excoriation. **Toddlers and preschoolers** develop control over defecation (toilet-training). **School-agers** and **adolescents** are self-conscious about body functions. Privacy and the use of a matter-of-fact approach to the subject is appropriate. **Young and middle-aged adults,** provided they are active, have little difficulty with bowel elimination. **Pregnant women** often develop **constipation** (passage of hard, dry stools) and hemorrhoids (distended blood vessels in the rectal area). **Older adults,** secondary to decreased activity levels and perhaps lack of water and/or fiber in the diet, are predisposed to constipation. To detect colon cancer, middle-aged and older-adults should be aware that a change in bowel habits and/or blood in the stool can be warning signs.

Clients must be **assessed** to determine if there are potential or actual problems with bowel elimination. Frequency (varies from person to person), color (brown is normal), and consistency (soft is normal) of stools should be determined. Changes from the usual pattern of bowel movements should also be noted (abnormal). The presence of abdominal distention (suggests constipation, excessive flatus, paralytic ileus, or intestinal obstruction) and bowel sounds (normal) should also be noted. Bowel sounds are absent with paralytic ileus (lack of peristalsis, often occurs secondary to surgery, anesthesia, immobility) or intestinal obstruction (below the point of obstruction) or excessive with diarrhea.

Nursing diagnoses pertinent to bowel elimination include the following:

- Bowel elimination, alteration in: constipation
- Bowel elimination, alteration in: diarrhea
- Bowel elimination, alteration in: incontinence

Planning and implementation for clients with regard to bowel elimination include teaching clients about the need for adequate intake of water and fiber and an active lifestyle to prevent constipation. The need to respond to the urge to defecate should be stressed. To facilitate normal elimination, privacy for defecation must be maintained, and an environment that is not anxiety-producing must be fostered. Personal bowel elimination habits should be facilitated as much as possible. Medications to encourage elimination of stool include cathartics and laxatives, and stool softeners. To help evacuate stool in a person who is constipated or who has a **fecal impaction** (hard stool that will not pass), an enema might be prescribed. Enema types include the **cleansing enema** (tap water, soap suds, and saline solutions that add bulk to the bowel, initiating peristaltic waves and bowel evacuation), the **oil retention enema** (softens feces to ease elimination of stool), and the **hypertonic enema** (Fleets enema, causes movement of fluid from the body to the bowel which causes distention of the bowel and evacuation of stool). Prior to some diagnostic or surgical procedures, a **high-colonic irrigation** may be required. **Digital disimpaction** may be necessary for relief of fecal impactions. **Bowel management programs** are often initiated for persons predisposed to constipation (include a combination of increasing fluids and fiber in the diet, maintaining activity, and perhaps stool softeners).

Flatulence (abnormal excessive air in the intestine, associated with painful cramping and abdominal distention) can be prevented by maintaining mobility and avoiding intake of gas-producing foods (cabbage, beans). Measures to alleviate flatulence include ambulation, alleviation of anxiety, abdominal massage, leg movement, insertion of a rectal tube, and administration of a **Harris flush.**

Diarrhea is usually associated with a disease process and can cause malabsorption, malnutrition, and fluid and electrolyte imbalances. Lost fluid must be replaced (preferably IV), food and fluid intake by mouth is limited and slowly reintroduced, and skin care at the rectal area is provided.

Incontinence of stool (involuntary expulsion of feces) is embarrassing and often associated with a disease process that interferes with nervous system control. **Bowel retraining** (establishing ar regular time for bowel evacuation, perhaps administering a suppository at a specified time) can be successful in resolving incontinence.

An **ostomy** is a temporary or permanent opening of the colon (**colostomy**) or ileum (**ileostomy**) onto the abdominal wall. Ileostomy stool is continuous and very loose, while stool from a colostomy is more formed and intermittent (especially in ostomies that are more distal). **Colostomy irrigation** is often useful in initiating a bowel movement at a specified time of day. People with ostomies require support in adjusting to a new method of bowel elimination and body image changes.

DRILL AND PRACTICE QUESTIONS FOR REVIEW

Complete the statements below.

1. The abnormal bowel elimination pattern that generally accompanies infection of the intestinal tract is _____.

2. An individual has surgery performed in which a loop of ileum is brought to the abdominal wall. This is called an _____. Stool will be _____.

3. In order to prevent the Valsalva maneuver when having a bowel movement, a person should be advised to _____.

4. A person who has had abdominal surgery may develop the bowel elimination problems _____ and/or _____ postop.

5. Bowel sounds are _____ with diarrhea. These are checked by _____ the abdomen.

6. A person with liver disease may pass stools that are _____.

7. A person with a bleeding gastric ulcer may pass stool that is _____ in color and _____ in consistency. This stool is called _____.

8. To determine if a stool that does not appear bloody contains blood, the nurse can test the stool for _____ blood.

9. A person with malabsorption passes stools containing fat. This kind of stool is called _____.

10. A person with dehydration is prone to the bowel elimination problem called _____.

11. A person is unable to control voluntarily the elimination of stool. This condition is called _____.

12. Including fiber in the diet is useful in preventing the bowel elimination problem, _____, and also helps to reduce blood _____ levels.

13. An adequate water intake for an average sized adult to prevent constipation is _____ cc per day.

14. To administer a soap suds enema, _____ml. of soap is added to 1000cc of water.

15. The most appropriate type of enema for a person with a fecal impaction is an _____ enema. This solution should be retained in the bowel for _____ minutes.

16. Under normal circumstances, when administering a soap suds enema, the client should be positioned in the _____ position. This position is useful because it _____.

17. The applicator tip of an enema tube is inserted _____ for an adult and _____ inches for children. The solution container should be held _____ inches above the bowel.

18. A high colonic irrigation may be prescribed prior to _____. For this procedure, an irrigation tube is inserted _____ inches for an adult.

19. A Harris flush is administered to relieve _____. It differs from an enema in that _____.

20. A nasogastric tube is inserted through the _____ into a person's _____.

21. A nasogastric tube can be used for _____ or _____.

Determine whether the following statements are TRUE or FALSE.

1. If a person has an urge to defecate, it will continue until defecation occurs.

2. A two-week-old infant passing four loose stools per day is in danger of severe dehydration.

3. A two-year-old child should be corrected for use of the words "number 2" when referring to stool.

4. A person receiving morphine is predisposed to diarrhea.

5. It is potentially dangerous to administer a tap water enema to a person with heart disease.

6. To prevent infection, sterile technique should be maintained when administering an enema.

7. Rapid instillation of enema solution is useful in preventing and alleviating cramping.

8. A warm drink is effective in promoting bowel elimination in some people.

9. A medication aimed at softening stool to ease bowel elimination is called a laxative.

10. Eating one large meal a day may help to prevent constipation.

11. A person with diarrhea is often placed on a diet that temporarily limits fluid intake.

Situations

Situation 1

You need to obtain a stool specimen from one-year-old Johnnie. List the steps you would take to obtain this specimen. In taking the specimen, you observe its black appearance. Are any further actions indicated?

Situation 2

Josie Smith is a seventy-year-old woman on bedrest because of a fractured hip. She has no other health problems except that she has not had a bowel movement in five days. Today, she passed a small amount of very hard stool. Formulate a nursing care plan (diagnoses, goals, criteria, interventions) for Josie relative to her bowel elimination problem.

Situation 3

Nikki Slomin is a client with intestinal obstruction. She has an NG tube in place. State nursing interventions relative to the fact that Nikki has an NG tube.

ANSWERS TO DRILL AND PRACTICE QUESTIONS

Completion Exercises

1. diarrhea

2. ileostomy, loose and continuous

3. exhale through the mouth

4. constipation, paralytic ileus

5. increased, auscultating

6. clay-colored or acholic

7. black, tarry; melena

8. occult

9. steatorrhea

10. constipation

11. incontinence

12. constipation, cholesterol

13. 2000

14. 5

15. oil-retention, 60

16. left Sims, allows gravity to aid instillation of the solution

17. 3-4, 2-3, 12-18

18. diagnostic or surgical procedure, 10-12

19. flatulence, tap water is instilled but the enema solution is instilled and expelled a number of times by raising and lowering the enema solution container

20. nose, stomach

21. administration of tube feedings, decompression of the GI tract

True/False Exercises

1.	F	6.	F
2.	F	7.	F
3.	F	8.	T
4.	F	9.	F
5.	T	10.	F
		11.	T

Situations

Situation 1

To obtain a stool specimen, do the following:
- wait until Johnnie has a bowel movement in his diaper
- don gloves
- use tongue blades to obtain and place a small specimen in a plastic or paper container designed for stool
- secure the lid of the container tightly
- label the container with Johnnie's full name and fill out appropriate requisition forms

Further actions:
- test a separate sample of stool for blood with a Hematest tablet or Hemoccult test
- notify physician of the abnormal stool color and test results

Situation 2

Nursing diagnosis: Bowel elimination, alteration in: constipation, related to immobility.
Goal: Josie will have a soft bowel movement every two days beginning the end of this week.
Criteria: Soft bowel movement passed without straining beginning the end of this week and at least every other day thereafter.
Interventions:
- determine high-residue (high-fiber) foods that Josie likes
- increase fiber in diet (fruits, vegetables) based on Josie's preferences
- offer adequate fluids (minimum 2000cc per day)
- turn Josie at least every two hours in bed
- encourage Josie to move her unaffected leg in bed as much as possible (e.g., ROJM)
- discuss with physician the possibility of a bowel-management program (use of laxative in conjunction with increase of fiber and fluids in diet)
- palpate Josie's abdomen to determine if it is distended from retention of feces
- observe Josie for passage of stool in adequate amounts
- recommend to physician the use of an enema or laxative if Josie fails to pass adequate stool

Situation 3

- ensure that tube is secured attached to the client's nose so that its position in the stomach in maintained
- tube should be attached to low, intermittent suction
- amount, color, and consistency of drainage should be observed, measured, and recorded
- patency of the tube should be checked periodically by temporarily disconnecting it from the suction source and observing for passage of drainage from the connecting tube to the suction apparatus
- irrigate tube as necessary to ensure patency (20-30 ml. saline)
- provide skin care to nares with water soluble lubricant to prevent breakdown of tissue
- provide mouth care (client will be NPO)

Chapter 47

URINARY ELIMINATION

NOTE TO STUDENT

The beginning of this chapter gives a useful review of the anatomy and physiology of the urinary tract. BE sure to refer to Table 47-1 for a review of the major life functions of the kidneys. The procedures in this chapter are of utmost importance to the nurse, and they should therefore be reviewed carefully.

MAJOR NURSING CONCEPTS

The expulsion of urine is called **voiding** or **micturation.** Examination of client's **urine** can give vital information about the client's health. The urine's normal characteristics, such as color (light yellow), appearance (clear), pH (under 7), and specific gravity (1.003 to 1.030) are important for nurses to know in order to compare with abnormal findings. Protein, ketones, glucose, cells, and occult blood are not found in normal urine. Conditions such as decreased blood pressure, stress, decreased fluid intake, decreased activity, and an increased secretion of antidiuretic hormone or aldosterone will decrease the amount of urine produced.

Urinary incontinence (involuntary loss of urine) is a common urinary elimination problem and is caused by many factors. The client with urinary incontinence requires meticulous **perineal care.** Incontinence during laughing or sneezing is called stress incontinence, and this client needs easy access to bathrooms, perineal **(kegel)** and abdominal exercises, and possibly surgery. Urinary catheterization is usually needed for **overflow incontinence** (when the bladder is full yet the person frequently voids very small amounts of urine and never empties the bladder). The client with **urgency** (an urgent need to void) also needs easy access to a bathroom. **Enuresis** (bedwetting) is caused by various factors, and various treatments such as bladder stretching exercises, medications, or psychological counseling are effective.

The inability to void **(urinary retention)** is a serious condition which may cause permanent bladder or kidney damage; it is treated with catheterization or medication **(cholinergics).** When urine is abnormally retained in the bladder after micturation **(residual urine),** it predisposes the person to urinary tract infections. Urinary tract infections are more common in females, produce symptoms such as urgency and burning on urination, and are treated with antibiotics.

A nursing **health history** specific to urinary elimination should include information about back pain, changes in urinary habits (excessive or diminished urination), **hematuria** (blood in the urine), frequency, urgency, and incontinence. Assessing for bladder tenderness and fullness, kidney tenderness, urine odors, redness (erythema) at the urinary meatus, skin crystals **(uremic frost;** indicative of kidney failure), and intake and output are nursing responsibilities.

Obtaining a urine specimen is often the nurse's responsibility. Many different collection devices such as external collectors (infant collectors, condom or Texas catheters, female collectors) are also used to prevent skin excoriation from incontinence. Urine may be collected by the nurse for a routine **urinalysis,** a **twenty-four-hour urine specimen** (the total amount of urine voided in a twenty-four-hour period), **double voided specimen** (client empties the bladder and urine is discarded; thirty minutes later a second specimen is obtained and tested), **first morning voidings, serial urine specimens** (to determine if there is an increasing or decreasing amounts of hematuria), and **clean catch** specimen (for urine culture). **Suprapubic aspiration,** which may be done by a physician or nurse, involves inserting a sterile needle through the abdominal wall into the bladder to obtain a urine for culture. Theoretically, this procedure produces a lesser risk of infection than catheterization does.

Nursing assessment often includes **urine testing.** Urine can be tested for glucose, protein, pH, ketones, and occult blood, using a test-tape or test strip. Simply dip the test strip into the urine, wait the appropriate time, and compare the color with the manufacturer's color code. Urine glucose may also be tested using the Clinitest tablets, and ketones with Acetest tablets. **Specific gravity** may be measured using a **urinometer** (need 20 to 30 ml. of urine) or a refractometer (need only one drop of urine).

A **nursing diagnosis** relevant to problems with urinary elimination is "alteration in urinary elimination patterns," which may include urinary retention and incontinence.

The **fetus** voids in utero at the fifth month. The **newborn** who does not void within twenty-four hours after birth is assessed for urinary tract abnormalities. **Infants** have no voluntary control of urination. **Toddlers** and **preschoolers** learn voluntary control of urination. Little girls should be taught to clean their perineums from front to back to reduce the risk of urinary tract infections. **Glomerulonephritis** (serious kidney disease which may result from a streptococcal infection) occurs is **school-agers** and is evidenced by dark blood in the urine and frequency of urination. Enuresis may continue during the early school years. The **adolescent** and **young adult** woman are at increased risk for urinary tract infection following sexual relations (often called **"honeymoon cystitis"**). The **middle-aged adult** male develops difficulty emptying his bladder because of an enlarged prostate gland pressing on the urethra or bladder, and medical attention should be sought. **Older adults** may have urinary problems (retention or incontinence) due to neurological deficits (stroke) or from their tendency to drink only small amounts of fluids (leads to concentrated urine and urinary tract infections).

Nursing interventions designed to promote urinary elimination include **bladder retraining programs** (for incontinent clients), providing **adequate fluid,** providing **privacy** (urination is considered a private act in our society), assisting with **position** (men may need to stand to void, and women to sit), and **relieving pain** (abdominal pain may interfere with urinary elimination). Additional suggestions are running water within hearing distance and making sure that bedpans and urinals are warm. Besides bedpans and urinals, a bedside commode (portable toilet may be used). **Diuretic** medications promote urine production by the kidneys, and **cholinergic** medications stimulate bladder emptying.

The purposes for **urinary catheterization** are for the removal of urine from the bladder, to determine the amount of residual urine, to decompress the bladder before surgery, to obtain a sterile specimen, and for bladder irrigation. If the catheter will be left in place after the procedure, the nurse will use a retention (indwelling or **Foley**) catheter instead of a straight catheter. Urinary catheterization increases the risk for urinary tract infections, may traumatize the urethra, may promote a decrease in bladder tone, and may pose a threat to self-esteem. The catheterization technique should be preceded by a full explanation and with the use of strict sterile technique and gentle insertion.

Nursing care of a client with a retention catheter involves possibly obtaining a specimen from the catheter, keeping the drainage container below the level of the bladder, taping the catheter to the client's leg to prevent accidental tugging on the catheter and possible dislodgement, checking frequently for kinks in the tubing which would impeded urine flow, and providing a leg bag for ambulatory clients. The urinary meatus of a catheterized client should be washed thoroughly with soap and water and rinsed at least twice a day. This washing is followed by an application of providone-iodine ointment. Gloves should be worn to protect your hands from body secretions. Intermittently irrigating catheters is controversial because of the risk of introducing bacteria into the urinary tract. If this procedure is ordered by the physician, it is to be done using strict sterile technique and equipment. Encouraging fluids (2,000 to 3,000 ml per day) is considered internal irrigation and is very effective. After the removal of a catheter, the client must be monitored closely for the return of normal urinary elimination.

Urine may be removed from the body by other methods such as **suprapubic catheters** (placed through a stab wound in the abdomen), **uretal catheters** (called **stints**), intermittent **self-catheterization, Crede** maneuver (manual expression of urine by pressing inward over the bladder), and **urinary diversions** (urotomy).

DRILL AND PRACTIICE QUESTIONS FOR REVIEW

Complete the statements below.

1. _____ is a bladder infection

2. An enzymelike substance which is produced by the kidneys and acts to raise blood pressure is _____.

3. An adult will accumulate approximately _____ ml of urine in the bladder before the urge to void is noted.

4. A diet high in _____ can cause fluid retention and decreased urine output.

5. Because women have shorter urethras, they are more prone to _____ than men are.

6. Perineal exercises involving intentionally starting and stopping the urinary flow are called _____ exercises.

7. When percussing the bladder, the nurse should know that a full bladder will sound resonant and empty bladder will sound _____.

8. Medications used to relax the urinary sphincter and promote urination are called _____.

9. Blood in the urine is called _____.

10. A Texas catheter is an example of a (an) _____ urinary collection device.

11. If one were interested in determining if there was an increasing or decreasing amount of blood in the urine, the appropriate test would be _____.

12. The specimen collection method used for urine culture is called a _____.

13. If you were using the Clinitest tablet method of testing the urine for sugar, you would place _____ of urine and _____ drops of water in the test tube.

14. A woman who develops a urinary tract infection following sexual activity is said to have _____.

15. Another name for an indwelling or retention catheter is a _____ catheter.

16. The standard size balloon in a retention catheter is _____ ml.

17. Periurethral care involves washing the urinary meatus with soap and water followed by the application of _____ ointment.

18. Internal catheter irrigation refers to encouraging _____.

19. Manually expressing urine by pressing inward and downward on the bladder is called the _____ maneuver.

20. A urinary diversion is also referred to as a (an) _____.

Determine whether the following statements are TRUE or FALSE

1. Urinary tract infections are potentially serious.

2. Erythropoietin is an enzyme produced by the kidney which stimulates the production of red blood cells.

3. Excess sodium in the diet may lead to renal calculi in susceptible persons.

4. Glucose and ketones are normally found in moderate amounts in the urine.

5. The alkalinity and acidity of the urine is influenced by diet.

6. Coffee and tea may cause urinary retention.

7. A major complication of urinary incontinence is skin excoration.

8. Overflow incontinence is not a major concern because the person is able to excrete small amounts of urine frequently.

9. Removing large quantities of urine from the bladder at one time may predispose the client to loss of bladder tone.

10. Urinary catheterization is done using sterile technique.

11. If a person is incontinent of urine, this fact should be documented on the intake and output record as "incontinent X 1."

12. Urine for a specific gravity test may be wrung from a diaper of an incontinent child.

13. Preschool girls should be encouraged to take bubble baths if they have urinary tract infections.

14. Automatic bedpan flushers and steamers sterilize bedpans.

15. Cholinergic drugs stimulate bladder emptying

16. The only problem with catheterization is the increased potential for urinary tract infections.

17. Foley catheters should be irrigated regularly in order to prevent urinary tract infections.

18. Another name for a uretal catheter is a stint catheter.

19. Strict sterile technique should be used for self-catheterization.

20. A person with a uretosigmoidostoy will excrete urine via his rectum.

Situations

Situation 1

Your neighbor, Mrs. Wittmann, tells you that her four-year-old daughter, Amy, has just been diagnosed with cystitis. The child's pediatrician gave her a prescription for an antibiotic. Mrs. Wittmann came to talk to you about Amy because she knows you are a nurse. List specific instructions you would give to Mrs. Wittmann concerning her care of Amy at this time.

Situation 2

Mr. Baker is hospitalized for renal failure. His physician has ordered a twenty-four-hour urine test for creatinine. List the steps you will take in order to obtain this specimen.

ANSWERS TO DRILL AND PRACTICE QUESTIONS

Completion Exercises

1. Cystitis
2. renin
3. 500
4. sodium
5. urinary tract infection
6. Kegel
7. flat
8. cholinergics
9. hematuria
10. external
11. serial urine specimens
12. clean catch specimen
13. 5, 10
14. honeymoon cystitis
15. Foley
16. 5
17. providine iodine ointment
18. oral fluids
19. Crede
20. urostomy

True/False Exercises

1. T		11. T
2. T		12. F
3. F		13. F
4. F		14. F
5. T		15. T
6. F		16. F
7. T		17. F
8. F		18. T
9. T		19 F
10. T		20. T

Situations

Situation 1

1. Remind Mrs. Wittmann of the importance of giving Amy the antibiotics for the entire seven to ten day medication regime.
2. Tell Mrs. Wittmann not to give Amy bubble baths now or in the future because they have been known to cause urethral irritation.
3. Tell Mrs. Wittmann to encourage Amy to drink as much fluids as she possibly can.
4. Be sure that Amy wipes herself from front to back after urinating or defecating.
5. If Amy develops back pain or a temperature, Mrs. Wittmann should call the pediatrician with this information.

Situation 2

1. Explain to Mr. Baker the need for obtaining this urine specimen and the need for his cooperation.
2. Then ask Mr. Baker to empty his bladder and discard this urine.
3. Document this time as the beginning of the twenty-four hours.
4. From this time and for the next twenty-four hours, you will collect all of Mr. Baker's urine and save it in a large container.
5. Refrigerate the specimens.
6. If any urine is inadvertently discarded, stop the test and start from the beginning.
7. Ask Mr. Baker to void at the end of the twenty-four hours and add that specimen t the collection bottle.

Chapter 48

WOUND HEALING

MAJOR NURSING CONCEPTS

Despite the cause of a **wound** (a break in the skin's surface), wounds normally heal in a predictable fashion in approximately seven days. Optimal wound healing (e.g., secondary to a clean surgical incision) is by **primary intention** (little scar tissue formation). Wounds that heal from the bottom up heal by **secondary intention** (some scar tissue formation); complicated healing (e.g., secondary to infection) is by **tertiary intention** (greatest amount of scar tissue formation).

The normal **stages of wound healing** include the inflammatory stage, the exudate or proliferative stage, and the regeneration stage. In the **inflammatory stage** (signaled by redness, heat, pain, swelling, and impaired function in the affected area), vasoconstriction, followed by an intense vasodilation and an increase in capillary permeability in the injured area, causes an influx of protective blood cells (leukocytes, platelets, erythrocytes, and antibodies) to the affected area. During the **exudative stage,** epidermal cells migrate over moist, healthy tissue (**granulation tissue,** which is very fragile and appears pink in color). Normal exudate may be serous (watery), fibrous (tacky), serosanguineous (blood-tinged), sanguineous (bloody), or catarrhal (containing mucous). Purulent exudate is abnormal and suggests infection. Eventually, cells in the injured area dry and form a protective seal over the healing area. During the **regeneration phase,** injured tissue is replaced with new functioning tissue (evolves from granulation tissue) or nonfunctional scar tissue.

Assessment of people for possible **wound-healing problems** is imperative. Poor wound healing may occur in persons who develop wound infections, and those receiving steroid medications, radiation therapy, or chemotherapy. People with poor circulation (e.g., diabetics) and those who have not been immunized against tetanus may also have complicated wound healing.

Specific **nursing diagnoses** related to wound healing include the following:

- Impaired tissue integrity
- Potential for infection

When **planning and implementing** care, measures must be instituted to encourage normal wound healing and prevent infection. Measures to promote normal wound healing include limiting tissue injury, encouraging blood supply to the area (avoiding restriction of blood supply; use of warm compresses), using strict surgical aseptic technique for cleansing of wounds and dressing changes, providing a well-balanced diet (with increased amounts of protein and vitamins A, B, and C), and limiting physical and psychological stress.

A **dressing** may be applied over a wound to protect it from microorganisms and injury and absorb drainage, although normal wound healing can occur without a dressing in place. If a dressing is used, the nurse independently decides to change a dressing (except the first postop

240

dressing) when it becomes moist or soiled or when it is necessary to inspect a wound (to determine if healing is normal or complicated) under the dressing (usually at least daily).

Cleansing of the wound and any **drains** (facilitate evacuation of drainage from the healing area) should be accomplished as necessary and/or as prescribed. Wound **irrigations** are sometimes ordered to help thoroughly cleanse deep wounds of drainage, debris, and dead tissue. Cleansing agents and irrigation solutions are usually prescribed, although the choice of dressing materials is usually a collaborative decision between the nurse and physician. **Debridement** (surgical removal of dead tissue) may be also be done to facilitate healing. It is important to note the progress of wound healing through accurate descriptions of the wound and drainage to other health-care providers, both verbally and in the client's record.

A **decubitus ulcer** is a specific kind of wound that is an area of necrotic (dead) tissue, caused by lack of blood supply to an area (usually secondary to pressure or shearing force). The sacrum, greater trochanters, and ischial tuberosities are most commonly affected. Decubitus ulcers develop in stages. In **stage one,** the area is initially pale but soon appears reddened but will blanch when touched. Eventually, a dusky appearance occurs. In **stage two,** the surface layer of skin ulcerates, and the edges appear inflamed. In **stage three,** dermis and subcutaneous tissue are ulcerated. In **stage four,** muscle and bone are eroded.

It is imperative to **assess** all clients for potential for development of decubiti. People at high risk include those who are immobilized, underweight, overweight, poorly nourished, edematous, and receiving pain medications. **Nursing diagnoses** pertaining to decubiti include the following:

- Impairment of tissue integrity, actual
- Impairment of tissue integrity, potential

Planning and Implementation activities related to decubiti include prevention of decubiti and care for decubiti. Prevention involves avoidance of pressure (turning, positioning, avoidance of shearing pressure, use of special pads or beds that reduce pressure), promotion of circulation (encouraging movement, providing massage around susceptible areas), and maintenance of skin health (preventing skin from getting too moist or too dry, avoiding linen wrinkles, providing a diet high in proteins, calories, and vitamins for immobilized persons). Treatment for decubiti involves increasing protein, caloric, and vitamin intake, and relieving pressure at the area. The area may be kept dry or moist (most recently preferred) with the use of semipermeable dressings. Debridement may be accomplished surgically or chemically. Treatment for decubiti is varied and controversial; many methods of treatment have proven successful.

DRILL AND PRACTICE QUESTIONS FOR REVIEW

Complete the statements below.

1. The signs and symptoms of inflammation include _____, _____, _____, and _____.
2. The process by which white blood cells destroy microorganisms is called _____.
3. Newly formed, pink, healthy, fragile tissue that develops in a healing wound is called _____ tissue.
4. Dead tissue is called _____ tissue.
5. The synthesis of collagen in healing wounds can be enhanced by application of topical Vitamin _____.

241

6. Bloody drainage is observed at a client's incision line. This is accurately described as _____.

7. A client who has had surgery healed with connected bands of scar tissue at the suture line. These are called _____.

8. A client with a cold is expectorating a lot of mucous secretions. This exudate is appropriately called _____ exudate.

9. Clients receiving radiation therapy or chemotherapy may heal poorly because these therapies _____.

10. Diabetics heal poorly because they have _____.

11. Persons who have had traumatic wounds should be checked to insure that they have been immunized against _____.

12. To facilitate healing of a surgical wound, _____ compresses can be applied to increase circulation in the area.

13. When performing dressing changes, _____ technique is indicated.

14. Necrotic tissue is surgically removed from an infected wound. This procedure is called _____.

15. Shiny, nonadherent dressing material is called _____. It is used when _____.

16. To relieve pressure on an abdominal suture line (especially in obese clients), a _____ can be used.

17. Nonabsorbable skin sutures are generally removed in _____ days.

18. The principal cause of decubitus ulcers is _____.

19. Decubiti are most likely to develop at the _____, _____, and _____.

20. A nurse pulls a client's skin against the sheets. This action creates a _____ force that can increase the potential for a decubitus ulcer.

Determine whether the following statements are TRUE or FALSE.

1. A client cuts his arm. It is normal to expect redness, swelling, and tenderness to be present.

2. A healing wound should be debrided of granulation tissue so that healing can continue.

3. Healing of a decubitus ulcer is optimal if it is kept moist.

4. To prevent pain associated with debridement, analgesics should be administered.

5. Wounds should be cleansed from outer to inner areas.

6. Sutures are best cleansed with the use of cotton balls.

7. Prolonged redness at an incision line may indicate infection.

8. Purulent drainage at an incision line is an indication of normal inflammation.

9. Stage 1 decubiti are the most advanced.

10. Placing a client in a wheelchair is similar to placing the same client in the supine position in bed.

11. To avoid shearing force, the head of the bed should remain at a 60 degree angle.

12. A rubber ring is useful in preventing pressure at the sacral area.

13. Semipermeable dressings such as Op-Site must be changed at least daily.

14. When using chemical debriding agents for decubiti care, the area should be cleansed well with tap water before application.

15. Heat application with the use of a goodneck lamp should be accomplished with the lamp placed at a distance of 12 inches from a decubitus ulcer.

Situations

Situation 1

Tracy Smith is a client who has had abdominal surgery. Her incision is infected and draining large amounts of purulent drainage that are currently soaking the dressing and tape. The skin around her incision is very reddened and excoriated because of frequent dressing changes and tape removal. Sterile gauze dressing changes are ordered. Wound cleansing with half-strength peroxide is also ordered. Describe exactly how you would position Tracy and why. State exactly how you would remove her dressing and dispose of it and why. State an alterate method of securing Tracy's dressing that would help prevent further skin excoriation.

Situation 2

Allen Kessler is a 12-year-old child who must stay in bed because of severe burns on his right arm (from fingers to below the shoulder), right hip, and upper leg. He is prone to decubiti because of his immobility. Discuss specific nursing measures to prevent decubiti in Allen.

Situation 3

Marcie Jack spends much of her day sitting in a wheelchair. What advice can you give Marcie to prevent decubiti formation?

ANSWERS TO DRILL AND PRACTICE QUESTIONS FOR REVIEW

Completion Exercises

1. redness, swelling, pain, heat, loss of function

2. phagocytosis

2. granulation

4. necrotic

5. A

6. sanguineous

7. adhesions

8. catarrhal

9. suppress immune system function

10. poor circulation

11. tetanus

12. warm

13. sterile

14. debridement

15. telfa, a dressing sticks to a wound and tissue is damaged when the dressing is removed

16. binder

17. 7-10

18. pressure

19. sacrum, greater trochanters, ischial tuberosities

20. shearing

True/False Exercises

1.	T	8.	F
2.	F	9.	F
3.	T	10.	T
4.	F	11.	F
5.	F	12.	F
6.	F	13.	F
7.	T	14.	F
		15.	F

Situations

Situation 1

Positioning:
- provide privacy by closing Tracy's curtain and/or door (Tracy's right)
- position Tracy comfortably in bed in the supine or low Fowler's position with breast and perineal areas draped (only appropriate position to visualize easily and work at abdominal incision site, respects Tracy's right to privacy)

Dressing removal and disposal:
- don gloves (protect self from infected materials)
- gently pull each piece of tape toward incision line (prevents pulling apart at incision)
- remove dressing and dispose of dressing materials and contaminated gloves in plastic bag (prevents contamination of others). **Note:** Since Tracy's wound is infected, she should be on drainage and secretion precautions, so the bag must be labelled and double-bagging should be accomplished after dressing change is completed
- montgomery straps would be preferred over tape (do not need to be removed each time the dressing is changed)

Situation 2

Measures to prevent decubiti in Allen:
- institute a turning schedule: reposition Allen at least every two hours (supine, prone, Fowler's, and left sidelying positions); the right sidelying position must be avoided; shearing force must be avoided when moving Allen
- apply lotion and massage around bony prominences: left shoulder, left elbow, left hip, right shoulder, left and right heels, and sacral area at least every four hours
- utilize sheepskin or foam pads at body prominences mentioned above
- provide a diet high in protein, calories, and vitamins

- obtain a pressure-relieving mattress or bed
- keep skin clean and dry
- keep bed free of wrinkles and crumbs

Situation 3

Marcie should be advised to do the following:
- lift herself off the seat for sixty seconds every half hour
- insure that the footrest is neither too high nor too low
- use a foam or water-filled cushion to reduce pressure at the ischial tuberosities

Chapter 49

ADMISSION AND DISCHARGE

MAJOR NURSING CONCEPTS

The change associated with admission or discharge from a health-care facility is stressful for the person involved and his/her support persons. **Admissions** may be brief (when a person attends an ambulatory or out-patient facility for nonserious illness or health maintenance care) or more prolonged (in-patient care, usually for serious surgery or serious illness care). **Triage** (immediate assessment to determine seriousness of a health problem and need for immediate care) is accomplished whenever a person is admitted for ambulatory illness care. Privacy should be afforded when health history and physical examination data are collected. Support should be offered when painful diagnostic testing is accomplished. The results of testing should be shared with clients as soon as possible. Admission for **ambulatory surgery** should include an orientation to the surgical experience prior to the day of surgery.

Admission for **in-patient** care (at least overnight) may involve admission to a nursing home, extended care facility, or a hospital. A nonemergency **hospital admission** usually involves a visit to an admitting department, diagnostic testing, transfer to an assigned room, orientation to patients' rights and new surroundings, introduction to staff members, securing of valuables, and identifying if a person has brought along his or her own medications (these should be sent home).

Assessment activities include a health interview and physical assessment to determine initial nursing diagnoses or problems. Baseline vital signs should be determined (initial measurements may be increased secondary to stress).

In **planning** care for children, growth and developmental stages must be considered. **Parental deprivation** can be psychologically damaging to children between six months and five years of age (children initially become angry, then withdrawn and depressed and decline in development). To prevent this, hospital stays should be as short as possible, parental visiting should be uninhibited, play and activity should be encouraged, a consistent care provider should be utilized, and adequate preparation for the experience should be provided. Adolescents and young children more easily adapt to separation but need contact with school activities and peers continued. Young and middle-aged adults usually find hospital admission extremely stressful in that it takes them away from family and livelihood. Older adults may fear death when hospitalized. They may also be fearful of the strange surroundings (often a new experience). Self-esteem and integrity may be threatened. In all cases, care should be individualized (likes and dislikes determined and respected). Safety and comfort should be insured. Data obtained from the client, response to admission, and procedures performed should be documented.

Discharge from a health-care facility involves planning to insure **continuity of care.** Planning for discharge should begin prior to admission to a facility. Discharge includes **assessment** to determine whether plans for care continue to be appropriate. If a person is being discharged to home and difficulties are anticipated, the **nursing diagnosis** "home management, impaired" may be appropriate. **Planning** for discharge may include referral to a community health agency for continued follow-up care. Continued care is necessary when physiological or psychological problems requiring guidance, teaching (of the client and/or support persons), supervision, or actual technical skills are present. A person in need of skilled nursing care is usually eligible for reimbursement of home health care services. Adequate support services are especially important for older adults.

A **discharge planner** is often available to assist with transition of care from an in-patient to an out-patient setting. In planning for discharge, activity restrictions or modifications, needed supplies (dressings, medications, IV's, etc.), diet prescriptions and meal preparation, and support persons must all be provided for.

Although most people leave a health-care facility with a written order of a physician, some leave against medical advice. In such a case, a person must be advised of potential health risks, but cannot be kept in a health-care facility against her or his wish. At the same time of discharge, verbal and written instructions for continued care should be provided. Any questions should be clarified. The instructions that are provided, client response to instructions, and arrangements made for continued care should all be documented.

DRILL AND PRACTICE QUESTIONS FOR REVIEW

Complete the statements below.

1. A client admitted to an emergency room for care is assessed by a nurse to determine the seriousness of the client's health problem. This procedure is called _____.

2. When a nurse makes an introduction to a new client, the nurse should tell the client his or her _____ and _____.

3. Vital signs immediately at admission are probably _____ than usual, secondary to the stress and anxiety of hospitalization.

4. Permanent psychological changes are more likely to occur in a child who is separated from a parent for more than _____ months.

5. A three-year-old hospitalized child begins to use a bottle again (had started drinking from a cup). This change in behavior is the result of a process called _____.

6. A nurse can most effectively serve in the role of substitute parent while a child is hospitalized by following a _____ staffing pattern.

7. Parental deprivation is more likely to occur in children from _____ to _____ years of age.

8. The _____ form of a drug is less expensive than the _____ form.

9. A client is generally transported to the lobby of a hospital for discharge in a _____.

10. A client receiving skilled home-nursing care is entitled to insurance reimbursement called _____.

Determine whether the following statements are TRUE or FALSE.

1. Ambulatory care is synonymous with out-patient care.

2. It is inappropriate to provide health education materials for clients to use in waiting rooms.

3. It is inappropriate to tell a client that his blood count is normal until a physician permits it.

4. Preoperative teaching for clients having ambulatory surgery is best accomplished the morning of surgery.

5. When a bed is being prepared for client admission, the bed should be placed in the low position.

6. It is not necessary to advise a person about patients' rights upon hospital admission because most people are aware of their rights.

7. A person in pain should not be offered comfort measures for pain relief until he or she has been seen by a physician to determine a medical diagnosis.

8. Planning for discharge should begin at the time of admission.

9. A community nurse referral is unnecessary if a support person will be providing care.

10. Health care is an obligation.

Situations

Situation 1

Tommy Williams, an 80-year-old client, is admitted to a hospital. He has no support persons with him. He is carrying $800 cash and three containers of oral medication. Discuss appropriate procedures for care of his cash and medication.

ANSWERS TO DRILL AND PRACTICE QUESTIONS

Completion Questions

1. triage
2. name, status
3. higher
4. 4
5. regression
6. primary nursing
7. 6 months, 5 years
8. generic, brand name
9. wheelchair
10. third party payments

True/False Exercises

1. T		6. F
2. F		7. F
3. F		8. T
4. F		9. F
5. T		10. F

Situations

Situation 1

Care of cash:
- money should be counted in the presence of the hospital cashier, the nurse, and Mr. Williams
- money should be placed in a sealed envelope which is signed by a cashier and by Mr. Williams
- a note should be made on the nursing-care plan (or somewhere in the client's record) stating that Mr. Williams's money has been secured in the cashier's office

Care of medication:
- the name of the medication and the reason for use should be determined
- Mr. Williams should be advised that he should not take his own medication while hospitalized
- medication should be taken from the bedside and stored in the medication area until Mr. Williams's discharge

Chapter 50

PERIOPERATIVE CARE

MAJOR NURSING CONCEPTS

Care for the client experiencing surgery includes **preoperative care** (before surgery), **intraoperative care** (during surgery), and **postoperative care** (after surgery). Whether surgery is performed on an emergency (life-saving) or elective (desired but not necessary) basis, and despite the setting (in-patient or ambulatory), the same basic principles of care apply.

Surgery initiates a stress response (vital functions are mobilized), disrupts the body's first line of defense against infection, interferes with circulation (secondary to blood loss), disrupts function of the involved tissue, and can threaten self-image and self-esteem.

Preoperative care includes a **preoperative interview** (conducted by nurse, physician, and person administering anesthesia) and **examination** and **diagnostic testing** to determine the **risk associated with surgery.** As part of the initial interview, fears associated with surgery should be determined. Clients at greater risk with surgery include obese clients (adipose tissue heals poorly and wound separation, such as **dehiscence** and **evisceration,** may occur; also, obese persons are less able to move); clients with nutritional deficiencies (especially protein, and vitamins C and D deficiencies, since these aid tissue healing); infants (surgery is more difficulty on smaller organs, fluid losses can be dangerous), growing children (must use resources for healing and growth), and the elderly (less able to deal with the respiratory and circulatory stresses of surgery); persons with cardiac or respiratory disease, diabetes (poor healing secondary to vascular problems), anemia (fewer red cells and oxygen for healing), kidney disease, infection (can spread to incised tissue) fluid and electrolyte imbalances; people with psychological problems or high anxiety; and those having major surgery (extensive trauma) or surgery involving vital organs.

Surgery is especially stressful for the parents of **newborns and infants.** The need for bonding must be acknowledged when surgery is performed on a newborn. Parental capabilities in providing care to newborns and infants must be fostered. The fear of abandonment and mutilation is strong with **toddlers and preschoolers;** therefore, orientation to the surgical environment and equipment and parental involvement throughout the perioperative experience are imperative. In general, postop recovery is quick with children. **School-agers** and **adolescents** often have misconceptions about surgery that must be identified and counteracted. Adolescents are especially concerned about body image. **Young adults** need to be advised that the fatigue they feel after surgery is normal. **Middle-aged adults** are often concerned about the possibility of a serious health problem (e.g., cancer). Often, surgery is necessary because of a health problem (whereas in earlier adult years, surgery is often necessary as a result of an accident). **Older adults** fear death with surgery and may delay surgery for this reason.

Preoperative teaching is an important aspect of preoperative care. Preoperative teaching should always be done, despite prior experience with surgery. Accurate information, in nonmedical terms, should be provided. Teaching should be done over a period of time, so it is not overwhelming. Demonstration and return demonstration of procedures that the client must perform should be carried out. Visual aids should be utilized as necessary. Support persons

250

should be included in preop teaching. Clients who have had a surgery similar to a particular client can provide information and support as part of preop teaching. Clients should be taught what will happen to them before, during, and after surgery and should be advised as to what they might feel. They should be told where they will be, what equipment will be used (they should see and touch the equipment), and whom they will come in contact with (personal introductions are helpful). **Deep breathing and coughing** exercises should be taught to prevent postoperative statis of mucous and promote optimal aeration of the lungs and oxygenation of tissues for healing. **Turning and leg exercises** should be taught to help prevent circulatory stasis and **thrombophlebitis. Informed consent** (surgeon's responsibility to tell the person about the surgery and all associated risks) must be obtained before surgery (from a client who is fully alert). The nurse is responsible for insuring that the surgeon meets his or her responsibility in fully informing the client and clarifying any questions or misconceptions.

Immediate preoperative care includes reducing bacteria on the skin at the surgical site (cleansing, hair removal), decreasing GI motility (NPO and perhaps enemas to prevent vomiting and constipation), and promotion of sleep and relaxation. On the morning of surgery, vital signs are assessed (abnormal readings may cause cancellation of surgery), and the client is prepared for surgery (dentures, jewelry, and prostheses removed; hospital gown donned; nailpolish removed; voiding accomplished; oral care provided; ID band secured). Special procedures are performed if ordered (NG tube intubation, foley cath passed, IV inserted, etc.). Preop meds are administered as prescribed to relax the client, prevent pain, decrease respiratory tract secretions (help prevent aspiration and pneumonia), and/or increase GI motility (prevent vomiting and paralytic ileus).

During the **intraoperative phase** of care, precautions are taken to protect the patient from physical and emotional injury and infection. Privacy and warmth should be maintained (hypothermia may occur secondary to environmental exposure and some anesthetics). Operating room personnel perform a **surgical scrub** and don sterile clothing to prevent introduction of any microbes to the client. A **circulating person** in the OR observes for and reports any break in sterile technique throughout surgery. The client is positioned to facilitate ease of incision by the surgeon (proper body alignment is maintained; and pressure on bony prominences, blood vessels, and nerves avoided). The client is anesthetized with a **general anesthetic** (depresses motor and sensory functions throughout the body, causes unconsciousness) or a **local anesthetic** (local effect, client is awake for surgery). An **encotracheal tube** is often used for administration of some general anesthetics and facilitates suctioning of mucous and administration of oxygen. Some general anesthetics are administered by the IV route. Fluid balance is maintained during surgery with the administration of IV fluids. Fluid balance is carefully monitored with use of intake and output measurements and other monitoring devices. Surgery can be performed with the use of a scalpel or a **laser** (an intense beam of light slices through tissue or binds it together), or **cryosurgery** can be performed (tissue is frozen and sloughs away).

Postoperative care generally involves immediate care in an area close to the OR (recovery room) and then later in an area where fuller recovery from surgery and anesthesia is accomplished. Immediately after surgery, a person must be observed for hemorrhage at the surgical site (obvious bleeding, pallor, low BP, increasing pulse), respiratory distress (snoring, gasping, restlessness, cyanosis, dyspnea), and pain. Positioning may be specified with specific surgeries or anesthetics (flat after spinal anesthesia). In general, a side-lying position is preferred to prevent aspiration of mucous or vomitus. Warmth should be maintained with the use of blankets as necessary. Vital signs are taken frequently. As the depressant effects of the anesthetic wears off, VS increase and the person is discharged to an area where recovery from surgery will be completed.

Throughout postop care, specific physicians' orders for positioning, etc., should be followed. Until the person is able to tolerate foods and fluids (gag reflex returned, bowel sounds present),

IV fluids will be prescribed. Intake and output should be monitored. VS should continue to be monitored until stable, and thereafter, to determine complications, such as infection (increase in temp and pulse). General comfort measures are important. Pain medication should not be withheld if necessary (BP and R should be checked to determine they are not too low for administration of a narcotic, however). As soon as possible, family members should be allowed to see the client. Breathing and coughing exercises, the use of an **incentive spirometer** (facilitates deep breathing), and turning and leg movement should be encouraged and initiated as soon as possible. Homan's sign should be checked to determine presence of thrombophlebitis. Medicating a person prior to exercise may facilitate activity and exercise. Normally, a noncatheterized person voids without difficulty after surgery (within eight hours). The first voiding should be noted and measured to make sure retention is not occurring. If a person does not void adequately, the bladder becomes distended, and backflow into the kidney can cause kidney damage. Measures to promote normal voiding should be initiated (having a man stand to void if permitted, running water, providing privacy, pouring water over the female perineum, and administering an analgesic to relax abdominal muscles). If necessary, a straight (one-time) or indwelling catheter may need to be inserted. Dressings should be changed, using sterile technique when they become soiled, and signs of infection observed (for prolonged redness, swelling, tenderness, purulent drainage, increase in temperature). The incision line and any drains should be cleansed as necessary. A binder should be used when a person prone to dehiscence or evisceration is OOB. Psychological support should be provided. Discharge planning should be comprehensive and include guidelines for a return visit for follow-up care, wound care, diet, activity, medications, and complications to observe for and report.

DRILL AND PRACTICE QUESTIONS FOR REVIEW

Complete the statements below.

1. Surgery that does not involve major risk and causes minimal trauma to tissue is called _____ surgery.

2. People with deficiencies of vitamins _____ and _____ are at increased risk with surgery because these vitamins facilitate wound healing. People with Vitamin _____ deficiencies are at increased risk of bleeding after surgery.

3. The presence of glycosuria may be a sign of the health problem, _____.

4. To determine if a person has kidney disease, the blood test, _____, should be performed on all preop clients.

5. A person with a low _____ count may require blood transfusions preoperatively.

6. Prior to surgery, a person can be taught the use of an _____, a device use to initiate a deep breath.

7. A person who has had surgery involving the _____ tract will probably need a nasogastric tube for decompression after surgery.

8. To decrease bacterial count in the intestine, patients having GI surgery are often prescribed _____ preoperatively.

9. Infants not receiving IV fluids should be NPO for no longer than _____.

10. A person is permitted to wear a wedding band to surgery if _____.

11. Elastic stockings should be applied with a person in the _____ position.

12. The drug Atropine is used preoperatively because it _____.

13. The drug Reglan is used preoperatively to prevent _____ and _____.

14. If blood is needed for a person during surgery, the _____ nurse is responsible for obtaining it and regulating the infusion.

15. A topical anesthetic is applied to _____.

16. Local infiltration anesthesia generally lasts about _____ minutes.

17. To prevent spinal headache in a person who has had spinal anesthesia, he or she should be kept in the _____ position for _____ hours and fluid intake _____.

18. Bronchospasm and larynogospasm are dangerous because they cause _____.

19. General anesthetics tend to _____ vital signs.

20. Operative blood loss can be determined with use of the blood test, _____.

Determine whether the following statements are TRUE or FALSE.

1. Chest X-rays are routinely done on persons of all age groups preoperatively.

2. It is likely that surgery will be cancelled if a person has a temp of 101 degrees F the morning of surgery.

3. Infants are especially fearful of mutilation with surgery.

4. The water pitcher should be removed from the bedside of an adult the evening before surgery.

5. Prior to surgery, people are placed on clear fluid diets.

6. Preoperative teaching should involve family members only if the person having surgery is a child.

7. It is inappropriate to tell a person preoperatively that he or she may feel pain postoperatively.

8. A person having major surgery should be shown equipment that will be used to monitor her or his fluid balance postoperatively.

9. The nurse is responsible for obtaining informed consent from a client prior to surgery.

10. Informed consent for surgery can be obtained from a sixteen-year-old mother.

11. Shaving of hair from the operative site is accomplished by shaving in a direction against the grain of the hair shaft.

12. A client who is NPO after surgery can be given ice chips.

13. Sleep medications should not be used by clients the night before surgery.

14. A person with a foley catheter should have the urine bag emptied prior to surgery.

15. Preoperative medications are generally given by vein.

16. Hypothermia commonly occurs with surgery and anesthesia.

17. A surgical scrub involves a ten-minute scrubbing of the hands and arms to 2 inches above the elbows.

18. During induction of anesthesia, OR personnel should maintain silence to prevent client injury.

19. The strings of a scrub gown worn by a surgeon are sterile.

20. A postoperative client should be placed in the semi-Fowler's position in the RR to prevent respiratory distress.

Situations

Situation 1

Mrs. Johnson is being prepared for surgery. Discuss the procedures you will teach her to prevent respiratory and circulatory complications postop. State the possible complications.

Situation 2

Shaun McGuire (16 years old) is recovering in the RR room after having received a general anesthetic for repair of an arm injury. Discuss nursing interventions aimed at preventing complications that might occur in response to the general anesthetic effects.

ANSWERS TO DRILL AND PRACTICE QUESTIONS

Completion Exercises

1. minor
2. C, D, K
3. diabetes
4. BUN
5. red blood cell, hemoglobin, or hematocrit
6. incentive spirometer
7. gastrointestinal
8. antibiotics
9. 4 hours
10. it is secured with tape
11. supine
12. dries respiratory tract secretions
13. vomiting, paralytic ileus
14. circulating
15. mucous membrane
16. 20
17. flat, 8, increased
18. respiratory obstruction
19. decrease
20. hematocrit

True/False Exercises

1.	F	11.	F
2.	T	12.	F
3.	F	13.	F
4.	T	14.	T

5. F	15. F
6. F	16. T
7. F	17. T
8. T	18. T
9. F	19. F
10. T	20. F

Situations

Situation 1

Respiratory complications:
- inadequate aeration of lungs and subsequent atelectasis (collapsed alveoli) and poor oxygenation of tissues
- stasis and accumulation of mucous and subsequent pneumonia

Circulatory complication:
- thrombophlebitis

To prevent respiratory complications:
- deep breathing (inhale through nose, hold breath a few seconds, exhale through mouth); perform five to ten times per hour
- coughing (if mucous is present)—in conjunction with deep breathing—after a few deep breaths with exhalation, forcibly expel mucous with use of chest muscles
- use of incentive spirometer
- splinting of the incision (support with hands and/or pillow) will help facilitate deep breathing and coughing

To prevent circulatory complication:
- turning every two hours
- moving legs through ROM as possible (flexion and extension) five times per hour
- use of elastic stockings

Situation 2

Nursing interventions:
- keep Shaun covered to prevent chilling (hypothermia is common)
- position Shaun on nonoperative side to prevent aspiration of mucous
- suction respiratory secretions as necessary to prevent respiratory obstruction and aspiration
- monitor VS to determine if dangerous overdepression is occurring
- avoid feeding Shaun food or fluids until ordered and until bowel sounds and gag reflex have returned (prevents vomiting and aspiration)
- position Shaun in proper alignment, making sure pressure on bony prominences, blood vessels, and nerves is avoided (Shaun will not be able to feel pain of tissue injury or respond as necessary)
- observe Shaun for suprapublic distention (depression of micturition reflex may occur)
- insure that Shaun is restrained on stretcher (prevents fall from lack of motor ability)